Balanced Choice

A Common Sense Cure for the U.S. Health Care Systems

Ivan J. Miller

Bloomington, IN Milton Keynes, UK

authorHOUSE®

AuthorHouse™
1663 Liberty Drive, Suite 200
Bloomington, IN 47403
www.authorhouse.com
Phone: 1-800-839-8640

AuthorHouse™ UK Ltd.
500 Avebury Boulevard
Central Milton Keynes, MK9 2BE
www.authorhouse.co.uk
Phone: 08001974150

This book is a work of non-fiction. Unless otherwise noted, the author and the publisher make no explicit guarantees as to the accuracy of the information contained in this book and in some cases, names of people and places have been altered to protect their privacy.

First published by AuthorHouse 9/1/2006

ISBN: 1-4259-5670-X (sc)

Library of Congress Control Number: 2006907237

Printed in the United States of America
Bloomington, Indiana

This book is printed on acid-free paper.

Dedication

In appreciation of Endaba Wilderness Retreat
and
its inspiration and help
in sustaining my energy for curing the health care systems.

Contents

Appendices

Acknowledgments

I could never have written this book without the support, encouragement, and ideas from friends and colleagues. They have worked beside me in many of my endeavors, stimulated my thinking, discussed the Balanced Choice ideas, provided suggestions, and contributed their own creative thoughts. I am fortunate that in addition to bringing me their good ideas, many of these friends and colleagues have also convincingly told me when I have bad ideas.

The prime supporter has been my friend and colleague, Lyn Gullette. She provided a writer's refuge at the Endaba Wilderness Retreat. When I was daunted, discouraged, overwhelmed, or feeling sorry for myself, she has reminded me that the ideas in Balanced Choice are important enough that I have to write the book. She has also been my primary editor, sounding board, and critic.

My family's backing has been essential. Maintaining a day job as a psychologist and an evening-and-weekend job as a health care reformer has been a strain on family life for 13 years. My wife, Millie, has learned to accept my hours of contemplation and preoccupation with health care, and she has remained lovingly supportive and encouraging. She has given important feedback and applied her artistic talents to all of the graphics and the logo. My grown children, Scott and Jon, have tolerated a father who often takes his computer on vacation, and they even appreciate my efforts to repair the health care systems.

For over 20 years, I have been a member of a discussion—writer's—activist group that meets monthly. Evi Bassoff, Wayne and Julie Phillips, Jed Shapiro, Lyn Gullette, and Dorothy Rupert have reviewed a painful number of iterations, and for many years they have encouraged my work, provided the necessary critiques, and made their own contributions to Balanced Choice.

My thinking about designing a better health care system began with my association with Karen Shore and the National Coalition of Mental Health Professionals and Consumers (NCMHPC). Karen was the first person I knew who tried to design a health care system, and she introduced me to the idea of gap payments. Two attorneys, Ken Anderson and Daniel Boone, taught me about monopsony, economics underlying health care, and the Sherman Anti-Trust Act. In addition, there are numerous members of the Board and local chapters of the NCMHPC who have stimulated my thinking.

The ongoing development of Balanced Choice has been supported and stimulated by the American Psychological Association, Interdivisional (39/42) Task Force on Managed Care and Health Care Policy—Mary Kilburn, Ed Lundeen, Stan Moldawsky, Stanley Graham, Bill McGillivrary, Gordon Herz, Joe Bak, Frank Goldberg, Russ Holstein, and Arthur Kovacs. In particular, Arthur Kovacs was the first person I knew who attempted to create a new health care system (Americare), and he provided extensive help with a major rewriting of Balanced Choice. He encouraged my work by believing in Balanced Choice and the notion that if a good system were designed, there would be a way to make it become a reality.

John Rifkin has been an earnest supporter and contributed the title of the book. I owe thanks to Chana Goussetis, Jonathan Miller, Hal Prink, Kathy Volker, Amy Kilbride, Christina Kauffman, Jim Bond, Gail Hollander, Ana Sanjuan, Don Marinelli, Wayne Adamo, and Karen Gray for reading and critiquing iterations of Balanced Choice. I owe a special thanks to Karen Gray for designing and creating the Balanced Choice web site.

I am grateful to Kathleen O'Conner for the audacious idea of having a national contest to develop a better health care system. The contest was encouraging and uplifting, and the opportunity to obtain feedback on an early version of Balanced Choice has been vital to creating the current version.

While I am the sole author of the book in a formal sense, Balanced Choice and the book are really the result of the ideas, support, and efforts of many, both those mentioned here and numerous others who have talked to me about parts of Balanced Choice. I am deeply appreciative of all of their contributions.

Preface

I am often asked, "How did a psychologist end up writing a book about curing America's health care system?" Thirteen years ago, I would not have imagined myself undertaking this kind of daunting task. Since 1993, however, I have been up to my neck in health care reform, advocating for consumers and providers in our broken health care systems. Early on, I decided that America was heading down the wrong path in health care, and I have been focused on finding another path. As the ideas for Balanced Choice have come together, it now makes sense that I should describe the other pathway. It also makes sense that the ideas needed to redesign the health care financing system would come from someone advocating for consumers and providers rather than someone in health care financing.

To answer the question about how I came to write this book, I think it is best to tell my story. Most of my life, I had wanted to be a psychologist, and, in 1986, I reached what I used to think was the pinnacle of my career. I received my Doctorate of Philosophy in Counseling Psychology from the University of Colorado. I had spent the previous 18 years working in mental health. My experience included working on the psychiatry unit at the University of Colorado Health Sciences Center. I learned about public mental health by working in the state psychiatric hospital, administering the hospital and hospital prevention services at the Boulder County Mental Health Center, and working for the Mental Health Center in all types of outpatient services. In 1986, I developed a private practice and became familiar with private-practice issues. At the time, I envisioned many years of satisfactory income performing the work I had always aspired to do.

My journey into health care reform began in 1993 when managed care began to dominate mental health care in Colorado. The success of my private practice was threatened by the gradual decline in referrals as the managed care companies began to control referrals to psychologists. Initially, I was unconcerned. I used my free time to take vacations with my family. I had heard that managed care was going to improve health care by rewarding those providers who were effective. I knew from my many years at the mental health center that I was good and efficient in my ability to obtain positive results, even with difficult cases. I was certain that managed care would want a therapist like me, and I was ready to join the managed care team. Although there were predictions of some cuts in pay, my needs were not extravagant, and I was sure that I would make a satisfactory income.

I signed up for a couple of managed care companies, and soon learned the reality of the managed care revolution. These companies had no concern about whether I was good or whether I was efficient. One of the managed care companies, Biodyne, obtained the contract for mental health services for one of my patient's employer. Biodyne invited most of the providers in the state to join its panel and come to its orientation meeting. In this meeting they administered a ridiculously simplistic test and had a brief discussion with six of us. The vice president conducting the interviews tried to calm our anxiety over the test and group discussion by explaining we had nothing to fear because everyone passed unless they were overtly psychotic. In essence, he explained that the interview and test were merely marketing gimmicks to persuade reluctant employers that their service was improving the quality of services by interviewing and testing all potential providers.

Under Biodyne, patients were told that their copayment would be drastically reduced while services would be improved. Having entered college on a math scholarship and having become proficient in statistics while obtaining my doctorate, I was able to add up the numbers that Biodyne was giving patients and providers. By looking at the amount it paid providers, the size of the copayments, and the estimated expense of its bureaucracy, I realized the only way that Biodyne could make a profit was to drastically cut needed mental health services. Later, I learned from James T. Wrich, an auditor of managed-behavioral-health-care companies, that financing the managed care bureaucracies was far more expensive than I had imagined, and that they did indeed have a need to cut valuable services. It became clear over the next few months that Biodyne required that providers learn to curtail treatment in exchange for possible future referrals. They ordered me to stop treatment on a long-term client in spite of the fact that treatment was clearly indicated and beneficial. The utilization review psychiatrist assigned to make me toe the line only backed down when I let him know that his dishonest behavior might result in a personal ethics complaint.

The reality of joining with managed care was different than the advance publicity. Instead of managed care companies operating through a genuine concern for improving treatment quality and efficiency, they showed interest in only two questions. Was I cheap? Was I obedient? While my fees might have been negotiable if the company had integrity, I was definitely not obedient when my integrity and honesty would be compromised.

This was a turning point for me. Many of my colleagues decided to work with managed care because they believed they could maintain integrity if they learned how to game the system, and/or they believed they could find ways to be honest with their patients in spite of the propaganda of managed care. It seemed to many health care professionals that managed care was here to stay and in control. It was not the same for me. Because of my understanding of math and numbers, it was clear to me that the managed care industry was not being truthful about what they could do for health care. To thrive as a managed care employee would have required compromising my integrity. I was heartsick about what managed care was doing to patients and the profession that I loved. I decided that I could not work within the managed care system.

The first steps down my new pathway were based on finding a way to maintain my private practice outside of managed care by increasing my number of self-pay patients. At the time, managed care was saying that it could provide mental health services for less money because it had discovered the power of ultrabrief therapy. I had analyzed enough research to know that ultrabrief therapy was a scam. I also knew that the mental health professionals in town were providing valuable services that consumers were willing to pay for out-of-pocket. As the ultrabrief therapy scam would come to be exposed, I believed there would still be a thriving market for mental health services outside of managed care. Time has proven this prediction true.

In the fall of 1993, I formed the Boulder Psychotherapists' Guild, Inc. to promote psychotherapy and the services of mental health professionals. With the help of several colleagues, I learned the principles of ethical marketing, and we talked 55 other therapists into paying $900 a year to join. This company is still thriving with 78 member therapists, and it has been replicated in a number of other locations. I am quite proud that this company is a model for ethical marketing. In addition, due to the Boulder Psychotherapists' Guild, I have been able to maintain a managed-care-free private practice.

As part of building the Guild, I realized that few people knew what was happening behind the scenes in the mental health marketplace. Consumers were unaware of how managed mental health care operated, and I decided to describe what was happening. I self-published a 50-page book *What Managed Care is Doing to Outpatient Mental Health: A Look Behind the Veil of Secrecy*, and I sold 5,000 copies. I also published a series of four articles in *Professional Psychology: Research and Practice[1]*, which exposed that the ultrabrief therapy model was based entirely on misquoted research. The actual research findings showed that using time limits to cut therapy short compromised the quality and outcome of therapy. That is not to say that there have not been many advances that are gradually making effective therapy briefer, but that the externally imposed limits that managed care was using compromised the quality and outcome of therapy. Dr. Harold Eist, President of the American Psychiatric Association, and I presented these findings at the American Psychiatric Association Convention in 1997, with commentary from four other mental health professional groups.[2]

At the time, mental health professionals all over the country were becoming concerned about the ethical compromises that were a result of the managed care system. The National Coalition of Mental Health Professionals and Consumers, Inc., was emerging as the leader of these professional groups. They discovered my book, and soon I was active on the national level as a board member and later as the Executive Director of the National Coalition. This brought me into contact with national activists in health care reform.

As I became involved in national professional politics, I realized that my life had profoundly changed. I have always thought that as a practicing psychologist I was doing my part to contribute to the world. My greatest goals had been to be a contented psychologist who might publish a few worthwhile articles. Now it was different. I discovered that I could make a difference on a larger scale. At the time, I was inspired by a leading psychologist, Dr. Arthur Kovacs, who at 68 years old talked of excitedly looking forward to how much he could do to make a better health care system by the time he was 80. Emulating him, I looked forward to the opportunity that I had.

I had become a leader as a spokesperson for integrity in mental health and for building a better mental health care system. I had improved my writing and speaking skills. Across the country, I had had the pleasure of meeting people who are concerned about the future of health care. Although I am not a traditionally religious person, I deeply believe in sort of a Stars Wars version of religion. I believe that by aligning ourselves with the Force of good, and staying away from the Dark Side, we can make a difference. I made a commitment to do my best to see what kind of role I could play in making a better health care system.

My experience working with the American Psychological Association and as the Executive Director of the National Coalition ended up shaping my decision to design a new health care system. Dr. Karen Shore, President of the National Coalition, and Dr. Arthur Kovacs frequently declared that, if we only tried, we should be able to design a health care system. This same thought resounded among professionals and consumers. Dr. Karen Shore introduced an idea she called Managed Cooperation. Her basic ideas are now part of the foundation for the Balanced Choice Health Care System. Dr. Arthur Kovacs was bold enough to attempt to design a complete health care system that he called Americare. Although both of these proposals had flaws, they inspired me to look for ways to overcome the deficiencies.

Meanwhile, I had opportunities to look at health care economics in a nontraditional way. My first exposé was a journal article written on the damaging effects of managed mental health care.[3] In this essay, I described how managed care could not save enough money to justify the enormous amount wasted on its administration and profit. In writing this article, I realized that by recovering the funds wasted by insurance and managed care there might be enough funds to finance a better health care system.

Some of my most valuable education about health care economics came as a result of my role as the Executive Director of the National Coalition. Our organization pursued a number of possible legal actions against the entire managed care industry, each of them focused on antitrust activities. In conjunction with Ken Anderson, a former department head in the Antitrust Division of the Department of Justice, we submitted a White Paper to the Department of Justice about possible antitrust activity and collusion.[4] The White Paper was followed by an interview with attorneys in the Department of Justice. While the political realities prevented the DOJ from taking an interest in these issues, I found the process highly educational. I learned about the basic economic underpinnings of the managed care industry at a level few people had explored. Most interesting was a similarity between managed care and monopsony, a dysfunctional economic system related to monopoly. A monopoly occurs when one entity controls all of the production, and a monopsony occurs when one entity controls all of the consumers. The similarity was that both managed care and monopsony took away consumer choice and controlled consumer behavior.

I realized that managed care and single payer systems were inherently flawed because both constrained consumer choices and, consequently, had diminished sensitivity to individual consumer needs. I was already aware that traditional insurance systems were flawed because they led to uncontrolled price escalation. In an attempt to correct the dysfunctions in these systems, I began looking for ways to develop a health care economic system that would restore consumer choices, allow providers to set fees, and have price competition.

In addition to studying the economics of health care, I have also had the opportunity to explore efforts to use science to improve health care. I was appointed to an American Psychological Association committee that established criteria for evaluating treatment guidelines. In other words, our committee's job was to come up with criteria for distinguishing good science from bad science. The goal was a set of criteria appropriate for all of health care, not just mental health care. The committee explored both the potential benefits of the evidence-based medicine movement and the potential dangers.

While developing a background in health care economics, I also devoted energy to consumer advocacy. Although I had found a way to practice psychology outside of managed care by serving clients who could pay out-of-pocket, this did not satisfy my desire to serve the broader public and those who could not afford services without assistance from insurance or the government. In Colorado, I was instrumental in establishing a Mental Health Insurance Action Line where volunteers helped consumers who encountered managed care obstacles to necessary treatment. The Action Line merged with a consumer advocacy group, the Patient Advocacy Coalition, which offered similar assistance for consumers with medical managed care problems. I became the Chair of the Board of Directors.

Through this work, I have become more familiar with the problems, efforts, and frustrations that consumers encounter with the health care mess. While our country is teaming with concerned citizens who are trying to repair problems in health care, these repairs are mostly underfunded band-aid approaches. These concerned citizens continually cite the need for a major overhaul. Their cries for reform are also continually stifled by the prevailing wisdom that fixing health care is either too expensive or that proposed solutions have too many flaws to obtain political support.

I have continued to wrestle with the idea that there must be a better way to design a health care system, and in the spring of 2003, I formulated my basic ideas in a proposal called Balanced Choice. Soon thereafter, Kathleen O'Connor created a national contest to find a solution for the health care crisis. She is a consumer advocate and health care analyst who has shared the frustration that so many have felt with the health care leaders. She also believed that there must be a way to fix the health care system and that the established leaders are not sufficiently aggressive in looking for solutions. She believed that the American people wanted an answer and that there were probably many people who had ideas that could help solve the problem. On a dare, she created the "Build an American Health Care System Contest" and called for submissions from any person in the country. All total, there were 109 entries and Balanced Choice was selected as one of ten finalists. After the contest, she formed a nationwide organization to advocate for fixing the health care system, Code Blue Now.

The feedback that I received after the contest indicated that this early version of Balanced Choice needed improvement. The judges did not seem to understand many of the concepts or the organization of Balanced Choice. The terms, explanations, and presentation needed to be clearer. I realized that it was not enough to figure out how to design a health care system; I also needed to describe the system in a manner that a typical college-educated person could understand it.

Experience in health care reform inevitably involves some time learning about the world of politics. In my early years of health care reform, I wrote a piece of model legislation that called for more transparency and disclosure from insurance companies. This "Consumer's Right to Know" legislation was supported by a coalition of all of Colorado's mental health professional organizations. It was crushed by the insurance industry soon after it was introduced. Several years after that defeat, I co-led another group that raised funding for the beginning of a ballot initiative process to take the same disclosure law to the voters. We eventually decided to abandon this endeavor because the effort required was greater than the amount the measure could contribute to making a better health care system. The lesson that I took away from these experiences was that a successful effort at health care reform would require a powerful coalition, which is why the Balanced Choice proposal is intended to unite consumers, professionals and employers.

With hindsight, I believe that it is not an accident that a psychologist could be proposing a way to cure the health care system mess. My background gives me the kind of overview that few others have. I have an understanding of science, economics, consumer advocacy, and advocacy for health care professionals. I have worked for public systems, worked for a quasi-public mental health center, run a private practice, run a small business, been an Executive Director for a nonprofit, worked on developing a potential antitrust lawsuit, been chair of the board of a consumer advocacy organization, spoken in twenty states about aspects of health care, been an administrator of inpatient and outpatient health care, and served on the front lines of health care delivery for 34 years. I may be in as good a position as anyone to come up with a novel solution, an outside-the-box approach.

Throughout the process of developing Balanced Choice, I have had the good fortune to have friends and colleagues who have encouraged me to develop my ideas. They have provided feedback, told me when my ideas are bad, and helped to develop the good ideas. In addition, they have reminded me that the ideas in Balanced Choice are so important that I need to disseminate them.

I intend to continue to promote and develop Balanced Choice, which I believe has the potential to be the best answer for curing what ails the health care systems in the United States. It has a better fundamental structure than other proposals, and it is inherently flexible, adjustable, and adaptable. I hope this book will gather support for Balanced Choice and help move the country toward curing the ailing U.S. health care systems.

Section I

Introduction to Balanced Choice

Chapter 1—Balanced Choice:
A Health Care Security System

The United States has nearly 46 million uninsured people. Many more people are underinsured, and still more fear the loss of their health insurance.[5] The problem does not come from spending too little money. The United States spends 47% more per capita on health care than does the next highest spending country, Switzerland, which, as almost every industrialized country, has universal coverage.[6] Measures of quality of care indicate that the United States ranks behind many industrialized countries—even those that spend less than 57% as much per capita as the United States.[7] Providers are dissatisfied with the enormous health care bureaucracy. The difficulties and restrictions of administratively complex insurance companies frustrate consumers. Employers can no longer afford the financial burden of health care and are cutting back on coverage. It is time for the United States to fix its health care systems.

Balanced Choice Health Care is a comprehensive plan that organizes health care delivery and the financing of universal coverage for an entire country—in this case, the United States. The result is a system that is good for the three important stakeholders— consumers, providers, and employers. For consumers, Balanced Choice is a system that is easy to use, allows choice, and gives the security of universal coverage. For providers, it allows choice about the degree of participation and, unlike a traditional single payer system, Balanced Choice does not impose government price controls. For employers, it reduces their portion of health care cost, and it ends their responsibility for providing health care coverage. Overall, Balanced Choice costs less than the current health care system.

Balanced Choice is innovative because it breaks through a fundamental impasse in health care reform. Reformers have been locked into two opposing camps, each with its own perspective. Each touts its advantages, but each also has essential weaknesses that prevent the development of adequate solutions to problems in the United States health care systems. Balanced Choice takes principles from each camp and combines them in a new way of organizing health care.

In one camp, proponents of single payer systems offer reforms that provide universal coverage. These proposals cost less than the current health care systems because they achieve tremendous cost savings by reducing administrative expenses. Single payer systems, however, involve government price controls that are unacceptable to the provider community. Moreover, both consumers and providers fear the loss of control over treatment decisions and the potential waiting lists that might occur. As a result, single payer systems, while preferred by many, lack the ability to overcome the political obstacles necessary for reform.

The other camp believes that improved coverage should come from a government sponsored expansion of insurance policies. This camp promotes the benefits of competition and the idea that government is smaller when health care is managed by insurance. Unfortunately, the proposals to expand insurance have several drawbacks. Expanding the number of people covered by insurance increases costs. Competition among insurance plans does not work well because consumers cannot predict their future health care needs or switch plans freely. Often, even with subsidies, consumers are unable to afford the insurance plan they need. Expanded insurance coverage would still have many gaps in coverage and leave people uninsured. When insurance companies manage health care, the result is bureaucratic restrictions on providers and consumers that are as onerous or worse than big government. Efforts to expand insurance coverage are stymied because these reforms increase costs and complexity, while still not providing universal coverage.

Balanced Choice offers the advantages desired by both camps. It balances two Plans—one Plan offers benefits very similar to a single payer system and the other Plan, based on market principles, offers more choices of providers. When balanced together, they provide a comprehensive, universal coverage health care security system in which both consumers and providers have freedom of choice. The entire system is able to achieve the administrative cost savings of a single payer system and also restrain prices. As a result, Balanced Choice costs less than is currently being spent on health care, and it provides universal coverage.

The system is described below, first from the consumer's perspective, and then from the provider's. Following the descriptions, questions are answered about how and why Balanced Choice works, how to overcome barriers to health care reform, and how the book is organized.

4

Balanced Choice System from the Consumer's Perspective

Choice of two Plans

In Balanced Choice, consumers always have two Plans—the Standard Plan and the Independent Plan. For patients, it is like having two health-care cards. The Plans have different payment arrangements. More providers are available on the Independent Plan, but, due to financial incentives in Balanced Choice, a good selection of providers is available in the Standard Plan. A patient may choose to use either Plan when selecting a provider, may see some providers on one Plan and some providers on the other Plan, and switch from one Plan to the other during the course of treatment with a provider. In other words, consumers decide which card to use each time they select a provider.

At first blush, it may seem undesirable to have two plans, but if the Standard Plan is high quality, it is no different than familiar situations in which consumers are perfectly comfortable. Grocery stores and restaurants have different tiers as far as quality is concerned. At a low cost supermarket, consumers can buy healthy and nutritious food, or they can go to an upscale market and obtain higher quality. Within a grocery store, there is often a discount brand and a higher-priced quality brand. Restaurants can range from inexpensive lunch counters to expensive five-star dining establishments. As long as consumers are not placed in a position of being limited to unhealthy or junk food, they appreciate the ability to make different decisions as various situations arise. If health care can offer a range of quality services at different costs, it could be a similar situation.

The Standard Plan

The Standard Plan is much like Medicare except that it is more comprehensive, includes a good pharmacy benefit, covers long-term care, and never pays too little to attract quality providers. To encourage early intervention and prevention of health problems, the first two visits each year to a primary care provider require no copayment. Other doctor visits require a small copayment. Patients make an affordable gap payment for medications and for some lab tests.

Guaranteed health care

No one needs to forego necessary health care due to an inability to pay. If a consumer is unable to pay, either because of low income or because of

5

a catastrophic and expensive illness, Balanced Choice covers copayments and gap payments. Providers are able to help identify patients with financial needs and can help initiate requests for assistance from Balanced Choice.

Emergency care

All emergency room care is covered under the Standard Plan so neither patients nor providers need to make decisions about which Plan to use in an emergency situation.

The Independent Plan

The Independent Plan offers the comprehensive coverage that is included in the Standard Plan but has both increased benefits and costs. The Independent Plan has a wider selection of providers and the providers may offer upgrades such as immediate appointments or longer visits. Balanced Choice pays a base payment for Independent Plan treatment, and patients pay a gap payment. Balanced Choice financial incentives keep the gap payments affordable enough so that patients will choose the Independent Side nearly half of the time.

Gap payments

Gap payments are an essential part of Balanced Choice. Gap payments are the difference (or gap) between a base payment made by Balanced Choice and the actual cost of a service. Base payments are set at a fixed amount for each type of service or medication, and the gap fluctuates as the cost changes. For example:

> Balanced Choice makes a base payment of $100 for an Independent doctor appointment. If a doctor charges $125, a patient pays a $25 gap payment, and if a doctor charges $135, a patient pays a $35 gap payment.

Lower prices

Gap payments are important because they lower the cost of health care for everyone by lowering prices. Cost-conscious consumers will look for lower prices. Consumers have control over the amount of the gap payment by considering the gap payment when choosing providers or various medications. Because Balanced Choice offers easy ways compare the size of the gap payments for providers and medications, the market pressure for lower costs is enhanced.

Costs less than the current system

Balanced Choice has significantly lower administrative costs than the health care insurance system. Balanced Choice has no marketing or advertising expenses. It does not need to pay stockholders. Balanced Choice saves so much money by lowering prices of health care and removing the insurance industry's administrative expenses, that it can provide universal health care coverage for less than the current expenditures on health care in the United States.

Balanced Choice System from a Provider Perspective

Choice of Plans

When accepting a new patient, providers decide whether to accept the patient on the Standard Plan or on the Independent Plan. Providers are always eligible to use either Plan. Each plan has a different payment arrangement.

The Standard Plan

In the Standard Plan, providers agree to accept the Standard Plan payment schedule. Financial incentives in Balanced Choice assure that Standard Plan payments are sufficient that providers, as a total group, willingly choose to accept Standard Plan patients over half the time.

The Independent Plan

In the Independent Plan, providers can charge more than the Standard Plan. Balanced Choice makes a base payment for each type of service and patients pay the gap between the provider's charges and the base payment.

Independent Plan providers need to offer something of greater value than the Standard Plan in order to have patients willing to pay the gap, which is higher than a Standard Plan copayment. Providers might persuade patients to pay Independent Plan charges because of a reputation for excellent care, specialized training or extensive experience. The justification could be improved service in the form of immediate appointments or longer visits.

Switching Plans

Providers may switch any or all patients from one plan to another. At any time, providers can switch an Independent Plan patient to the lower cost Standard Plan. This might happen if the provider wished to retain a long-term patient who encountered financial hardships and could no longer pay the Independent Plan gap payments. Providers may switch an established Standard Plan patient to the more costly Independent Plan by giving the patient a one-year's advance notice. Providers are also free to raise Independent Plan fees if they give adequate notice to current patients.

Market forces determine reimbursement rates

The reimbursement rates for the Standard Plan and the Independent Plan are both responsive to market forces. If Standard Plan reimbursements are below market expectations, enough providers will discontinue taking new Standard Plan patients, and Balanced Choice is mandated to increase Standard Plan reimbursements. If Independent Plan reimbursements are too low, the gap payments will become so large that consumers will refuse to use the Independent Plan. As a result, providers will need to lower Independent Plan fees.

Reduced operating expenses and improved job satisfaction

Balanced Choice reduces providers' operating expenses and improves job satisfaction. Providers no longer need to maintain large administrative staffing to deal with multiple insurance plans. Since all patients are covered, providers do not need to worry about patients' lack of insurance, changes in insurance, or managed care restrictions. Managed care is greatly reduced. Instead of devoting time to relationships with insurance companies, providers are free to focus on the provider-patient relationship.

Questions and Answers about Balanced Choice

Why should Balanced Choice work better than single payer or insurance?

Balanced Choice is based on fundamentally different economic principles than either a single payer or insurance-based system. Although health care economics seems daunting to many people, the basic principles in each of the systems are not difficult to understand. Chapter 2, "Making Sense of Health Care Economics," explains how problems in health care are caused by the economic shortcomings of insurance, single payer, and managed care. Based on this explanation, Chapter 3, "Balanced Choice: A Functional Market System," describes how Balanced Choice overcomes the economic weaknesses in other financing systems. These two chapters are key to understanding how and why Balanced Choice is a better way to fix the health care system.

How will the Standard Plan be prevented from evolving into substandard care for the poor?

Many health care advocates have avoided a two-tiered system for fear that the lower tier would be starved of funding and gradually deteriorate into substandard care for the poor. Balanced Choice has an innovative mechanism, the Mandatory Funding Split, that corrects for the tendency for the Standard Plan to deteriorate. This mandated split assures that the Standard Plan always receives a large-enough portion of the funding that it cannot be starved of funds. As explained in detail in Chapter 3, "Balanced Choice: A Functional Market System," this Mandatory Funding Split keeps the Standard Plan and Independent Plan in balance. As a result the Standard Plan is always seen as a reasonable way for the majority of consumers to obtain quality health care and as an acceptable way for the majority of providers to receive payment for services.

How will Balanced Choice be financed?

Balanced Choice proposes obtaining funding, as much as possible, from monies that are currently being spent on health care. All state and federal funds that are currently allocated for health care would be transferred to Balanced Choice. Employers' current contributions to health care insurance would be diverted to a Balanced Choice Health Care Fund in the new system, with an overall savings for employers of $100 billion annually. Likewise, employees' contributions to health insurance would be replaced by contributions to the Balanced Choice Health Care Fund based on a percentage of their earnings. Chapter 4, "An Outline for Financing Balanced Choice," explains the financing proposal.

How does Balanced Choice impact employers?

In Balanced Choice, employers are no longer responsible for health care. They no longer need to select or manage benefit packages and none of the employer's staff or the employee's working time is devoted to learning, understanding and managing insurance plans. Employers are freed also from the responsibility for paying for the health care portions of workers' compensation and auto insurance. In other words, they no longer have responsibility for managing health care coverage.

Employers' overall expenses for health care are lowered. Balanced Choice is partially funded by an employer's contribution to a Balanced Choice Health Care Fund, but this *increase would be $100 billion less than the overall annual amount employers already spend on health insurance.* This financial contribution will not increase as health care costs increase. If more funds are needed for future health care, they will need to come from other revenue sources, not employers. Instead of being faced with rising health care costs and workers' compensation costs, employers will obtain immediate relief and have a responsibility only for a predictable portion of their payroll.

Employers who have not been paying for health care will be protected from the hardship of having to contribute to the Balanced Choice Health Care Fund. These employers will have their contributions to the Balanced Choice Health Care Fund added at less than the rate of annual inflation.

In addition to savings on the expense of providing employees health care, employers would obtain a savings from workers' compensation insurance and automobile insurance. Because all health care would be covered in Balanced Choice, health related expenses in workers' compensation and automobile insurance would not be necessary.

Once employers are freed of responsibilities for health care, they can do what they do best—focus on business. In addition to lowered direct costs, they will have the indirect benefit of eliminating all the time that management of health care has diverted from productivity. Balanced Choice will enhance the ability of American business to compete in the global marketplace.

Is Balanced Choice complicated to use?

Balanced Choice is far easier to use than managed care or most insurance. Although Balanced Choice calls for a shift in thinking about health care, Balanced Choice makes choices and costs so clear that health care is no more complex than familiar areas of the economy. Chapter 5, "The Consumer-Friendly Experience in Balanced Choice," and Chapter 6, "The Provider-Friendly Experience in Balanced Choice," describe the daily experience of Balanced Choice from the perspective of consumers and providers respectively. Chapter 7, "A Balanced Choice Pharmacy Plan," describes how a Balanced Choice system could create a Medicare Pharmacy Benefit system that is much easier and more efficient than the current Medicare pharmacy program.

Does Balanced Choice improve health care?

Balanced Choice has a proposal for encouraging the improvement of health care through the use and development of evidence-based medicine, which is described in Chapter 8, "Science, Education, and Consumer Advocacy." Chapter 9, "More Features and Innovation," describes how Balanced Choice encourages prevention services, provides incentives for underserved communities, provides long-term care, reduces malpractice insurance, consolidates information on public health and health care trends, and is open to a broad array of cost-containment strategies when appropriate.

Are there other proposals that accomplish the goals of Balanced Choice?

The other proposals do not solve the problems of health care financing as well as Balanced Choice. Chapter 10, "Health Care Insurance is Obsolete," explains why traditional insurance actually causes many of the problems in health care financing. Insurance-based proposals are too expensive to implement, and Chapter 11, "Patching-up Insurance-Driven Health Care," explains the ways that Balanced Choice is superior to insurance-based proposals. Single payer proposals are not politically feasible, and Chapter 12, "Single Payer Compared to Balanced Choice," explains the ways Balanced Choice is better than a single payer system.

Can such an innovative system work?

Skeptics might raise a number of questions about Balanced Choice. Can consumers take a responsible role in health care decisions? Can market forces slow the rising cost of health care? Are the innovations too complicated? Chapter 13, "Solid Advantages with Balanced Choice: A Reply to Skepticism," examines these questions and argues that there is good reason to believe that Balanced Choice is a solid program that not only can work, but works better than the alternative proposals.

How does Balanced Choice need to be developed?

Balanced Choice is a flexible and evolving proposal. As feedback develops, the system can be modified. Research, modeling, and cost estimates need to be conducted. Chapter 14, "Traveling the Road to the Cure: Consumers, Providers, and Employers Lead," describes areas that need further development.

Can insurance industry opposition be overcome?

A barrier to Balanced Choice is opposition from the insurance industry. A common reaction to Balanced Choice is skepticism that any proposal can be advanced if it does not include the insurance industry. Indeed, many people in the expand-insurance camp cite this belief as the primary reason they are supporting expanding insurance through government subsidies.

Overcoming the opposition from insurance may not be as impossible as feared. Balanced Choice accomplishes the goals that the insurance industry promotes—restraining costs while offering choice. In fact, the insurance industry is increasingly using methods similar to Balanced Choice. Obtaining near universal coverage with insurance would be much more expensive and complicated than with Balanced Choice. If Balanced Choice were in the discussion of the best way to fix the health care systems, there would be tremendous pressure from consumers, providers, and employers to use a system that is simpler and less expensive. The combined political pressure from consumers, providers, and employers, once they understand how much simpler and less expensive Balanced Choice is, makes overcoming the resistance of the insurance industry possible.

Is Balanced Choice too drastic a solution?

A complete overhaul of the U.S. health care systems is needed. Such an overhaul is drastic. Balanced Choice is drastic, but less drastic proposals would not be as effective or efficient.

Is Balanced Choice too good to be true?

It is not that Balanced Choice is too good to be true, but that the current insurance-driven and managed care system is so bad that there is plenty of money for a sensible system. After all, the U.S. has the most expensive system in the world, 46 million uninsured, and only mediocre outcomes compared to other industrialized countries. Balanced Choice would merely provide the quality, accessibility, and efficiency that the U.S. deserves considering how much is already being spent on health care.

What steps will make Balanced Choice an option for health care reform?

Balanced Choice is a combination of common-sense ideas, which create a new outside-of-the-box solution. As with all new ideas, they cannot be considered until they are articulated and described. Therefore, one of the first steps in making Balanced Choice an option for health care reform is writing this book, so that readers can examine a comprehensive description of the combination of ideas that are referred to as Balanced Choice.

Once the ideas in Balanced Choice are described, the goal is to have the ideas become well known enough to be considered as a reform proposal. The established channels for reform, however, will only slowly be opened to a new proposal.

The health care industry is unlikely to be an early source of support for ideas that reorganize health care and health care financing. While the problems of health care are well known, it is important to recognize that the health care industry is not having a crisis. The enormous amount being spent on health care is a bonanza for the health care industry. The big players—pharmaceutical companies, insurance companies, and hospital corporations—are doing very well. Overall, the health care industry is thriving.

The proponents of health care reform are in two opposing camps. Neither camp is looking for a proposal that incorporates features of the other one. Professional and consumer organizations need to maintain their alliances with both camps, and they cannot afford to spend their political capital on a new and virtually unknown proposal that might alienate them from advocates of the established camps. Politicians cannot risk supporting a little-known idea that does not yet have an established constituency.

Support for a system that combines features from both camps is most likely to come from the groups that are experiencing the health care crisis—consumers, providers, and employers, who are the intended audience for this book. Consumers want a system that has the security of single payer with the option of paying more for improved services. Providers want a system that is simple, provides comprehensive care, and does not impose rigid price controls. Employers want relief from the burden of health care financing. Balanced Choice meets their needs better than other proposals.

One avenue for advancing Balanced Choice is making it a popular and familiar option that gradually develops grassroots support from consumers, providers, and employers. The other avenue is to have it available as an option when health care reform becomes more necessary. As change becomes more likely, there will be more pressure for compromise—for a proposal that combines the benefits from each camp and overcomes the weaknesses of each camp. If Balanced Choice is a recognized option, it may become the solution that the United States needs.

Section II

Economics
and Balanced Choice

Chapter 2—Making Sense
of Health Care Economics

Summary: Understanding how Balanced Choice cures the United States health care systems begins with making sense of health care economics. A simple free market does not work because health care is too expensive for most ill people to afford. In order to provide limited health care security, insurance has become the dominant health care financing system. Insurance-driven health care results in price escalation because, when insurance was paying the bills, neither consumers nor providers were concerned about how much health care costs. To control price escalation, managed care was created, but it is disliked by consumers and providers and creates its own problems with the quality and accessibility of health care. A proposed alternative to insurance and managed care, a single payer system, creates fears of government price controls and also has potential problems with maintaining quality and accessibility. Each of these economic systems has underlying dysfunctions, and a better system is needed.

Where did the United States health care systems go wrong? What are the choices for the future? How can health care get back on the right road? Understanding what went wrong and how it can be fixed requires making sense of the health care economics that underlie each health care financing system.

A Free Market

Before World War II, most health care was financed based on the principles of a simple free market. People were expected primarily to fend for themselves and to pay for any health care expenses that arose. Expenses were not that great and health insurance was uncommon. The wealthy could pay for health care, but others often needed to rely on charity or public hospitals that had substandard care.

The simple free market is no longer a viable option. Many modern treatments are just too expensive for most people to afford. Chronic illnesses can be catastrophically expensive. Savings can be wiped out by the unpredictable misfortunes of an accident, illness, or health condition. Returning to a free market would result in health care insecurity for all but the wealthiest families. A compassionate society wants a health care system that is good for everyone, not just the fortunate.

Although the free market is no solution for financing health care, it is, when functioning well, the model for a healthy economic system. Undeniably, there are many areas of the economy where a free market functions well. Balanced Choice's goal is to create a health care system that functions as well as the free market system does in other areas of the economy. Understanding a well-functioning free market is a good place to start in understanding health care economics.

The well-functioning free market has three dynamics. First, competition presses for *lower prices*. Second, in order to meet the demand of consumers, competitors make goods and services readily available and accessible. And third, competition *raises the quality* of goods and services. When systems work properly, the amazing result is something that every consumer can easily identify—lower prices, higher quality, and easy availability or accessibility.

Properly Functioning Free Market Dynamics

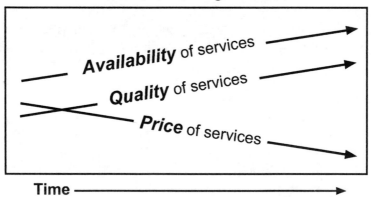

These dynamics are apparent to consumers in the choices that they make in their everyday shopping. When making purchases, whether for groceries, clothing, or electronic equipment, consumers ask three basic questions. What's the price? How good is the quality? And, what is available at each store? Sometimes when price is most important, consumers go to a discount store; when availability is more important they go to the most convenient store; and when quality or personal service is important they might go to a specialty store.

Providers know that they can charge more by improving the quality or the availability of their services. They can also lower prices to increase their volume of business. Quality services and enterprising activity are rewarded in such a system.

The Insurance-Driven Health Care System

In World War II, due to an accident of history, employers began paying for health care insurance.[8] Because of a federally mandated wage freeze, employers could not attract new employees with higher salaries. To compete for desperately needed employees, they began offering fringe benefits, which were exempt from the wage freeze. These fringe benefits included health insurance. America began its tradition of having employers take a primary role in providing health care.

Since its beginning during World War II, insurance-driven health care has become the dominant way of financing health care. In the doctor's office, often the first question following, "What is your name?" is, "What is your insurance company?" Currently, some insurance is provided by employers, some is purchased by individuals, and some is funded by the government. Most people have come to believe that having traditional insurance is the only way they can have health care security. Indeed, until the 1980s, when health care cost escalation forced the movement to managed care, insurance-driven health care was a good option.

In many parts of the economy, insurance functions well. When insurance works, it spreads the risk of a catastrophic event. Take for instance, the possibility that fire could burn someone's home. This might happen to one out of a thousand people. If all thousand people pool a small amount of their money in an insurance company, when the one-in-a-thousand homes burns to the ground, there is money to rebuild the home. This is the legitimate business of insurance—spreading the risk of a large unfortunate event.

In health care, insurance is different than in other areas of the economy. It not only spreads the risk of a catastrophic event, but also is now considered the way to pay for most health care expenses. Doctor's visits, medications, and routine lab tests are paid by insurance as well as the costs of catastrophic illness. Instead of merely spreading the financial risk of catastrophic medical expenses, insurance became a prepayment system that covers all health care.

Because health insurance pays for most care, it has created a major problem in market dynamics. Insurance coverage has caused consumers to lose their cost consciousness. If people have insurance, they often say, "I don't care how much it costs, insurance is paying the bill." When most of the people say cost does not matter, fees escalate unreasonably—no one is comparing prices like they do in a healthy market system. This loss of cost-consciousness is generally considered to be the cause of the price escalation in health care before the advent of managed care.

In insurance-driven health care, patients ask for the highest quality care and readily available care. Thus there are market dynamics that improve quality and accessibility. The consequence of insurance-driven health care is a rapidly growing, high-quality health care system with great accessibility to a patient's chosen provider. But, as mentioned above, the dynamics lead to an excessive rise in costs that is unsustainable.

Insurance-Driven Market Dynamics

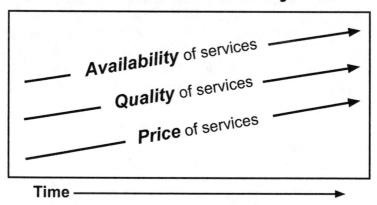

Understanding how insurance does *not* work for financing health care is essential to curing the system. When insurance sticks to the business of insurance, spreading the risk of a catastrophic event, prices in the marketplace are not affected. To return to the example of the one-in-a-thousand homes burning down, the cost of new homes in general does not go up just because the family rebuilding the burned home says, "We don't care how much it costs because insurance is paying the bill." The cost of homes and repairs, as well as homeowner insurance would increase unreasonably if homeowner insurance paid for all home related expenses the way that health insurance pays for all health related expenses.

This problem can be further clarified by imagining what car insurance would be like if it were used to finance all expenses related to automobiles. Insurance would pay for gasoline, oil changes, new tires, and repairs, in addition to major accidents. Not only would the insurance cost be enormous, but also the cost of routine items—gasoline, tires, oil changes, new tires, and repairs—would rise sharply, as consumers would say, "I don't care how much it costs because insurance is paying the bill." Quality would rise and the availability of services would improve, as consumers would want high quality and convenient access. Soon, the cost of automobile insurance would be out of sight. Due to the high cost of automobile-related expenses, many consumers would be unable to afford to operate a car without insurance, and often unable to afford the insurance.

Managed Care: An Attempt To Fix Insurance-Driven Health Care

In the 1980s, double-digit inflation in health care caused the nation to realize that insurance-driven health care systems were unsustainable. Consumers had lost cost consciousness, and price escalation of insurance was unbearable for employers. The attempted solution was to add managed care. Because conventional wisdom had abandoned the idea of restoring cost consciousness in consumers, it was incorrectly assumed that managed care was the answer. It has now become the dominant form of health care in the United States. Managed care, unfortunately, continues to undermine cost consciousness by promising consumers that their only financial responsibility is to make small copayments.

Although managed care temporarily contained price escalation, it created its own set of problems. It is extraordinarily expensive to operate. It requires organizing an extensive network of providers and developing bureaucratic systems to control the providers. Although it has been successful at cutting costs, it has accomplished this by compromising quality and accessibility.

One needs to use imagination to think of an example of an economic system similar to managed care. Imagine having groceries managed. In the managed grocery system, employers would assign their employees to a grocery store that decided how much food and what kind of food each member could consume. The store would use secret proprietary policies to determine which foods were worth the cost. Consumers would make a flat copayment each time that they went to the grocery store.

Undoubtedly, these managed grocery stores could provide nutritious food for all of the members. Indeed, these stores could prevent people from gluttony and poor food choices. Starvation would not be a concern because of government regulation and the public outrage that would result if the managed grocery store did not feed its members. However, it is doubtful that these privately managed grocery stores, each striving to lower costs and increase profits to shareholders, would provide the abundant and plentiful quantities of choices that are available in the current free market grocery stores.

Managed care operates differently than the large group or cooperative, which obtains lower costs with their purchasing power. In a cooperative or group purchase, consumers are free to use the cooperative or to purchase goods and services elsewhere. In order for managed care to have enough power to lower prices to the degree necessary in health care, it also needs control over consumer health care decisions. It tells consumers which providers can be seen and what services will be covered.

Managed Care Dynamics

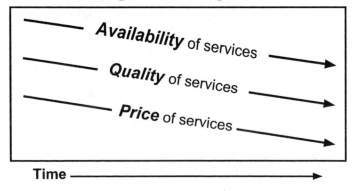

While managed care is powerful in cutting medical costs (the added costs of administration, marketing, and profit-taking are discussed elsewhere), it creates unhealthy market dynamics. Once consumer choice is gone, providers are no longer solely responsive to patients and are pressured to serve the managed care company. Managed care companies have earned a reputation for creating barriers, hassles, and frustrations that prevent patients from obtaining high-quality treatment, and that restrict the availability of providers.

How does managed care hurt quality and accessibility?

Market-based managed care advocates hoped that managed care would merely lower costs reasonably without also lowering quality or undermining accessibility. Managed care has not achieved this ideal, and for several reasons, it does not seem possible that it ever could. First, it is much easier to measure cost than changes in quality or accessibility. Those who operate managed care, even if well intentioned, can always demonstrate a savings in cost even if it is only a penny. They cannot, on the other hand, quantify the impact of small changes in the intangible aspects of quality or accessibility. Difficulties finding an acceptable or compatible doctor, the subjective feelings of discomfort, or the bedside manner of providers are not as measurable as money. The result is that cost trumps quality and accessibility. Second, the managed care companies do not have interests aligned with patients. The officers of managed care companies care more about pleasing stockholders than maximizing the health of patients. Third, a managed care company needs to make decisions for the typical patient, and as a result, errs in the tendency to select one size to fit all.

Managed care companies are aware of their potential negative impact on health care, and propose complex mechanisms to maintain quality. They suggested that scientific and computer analysis of outcomes would be used to assure that managed care companies compete to have the highest quality services and the best access to services. While computers and science are wonderful, the complex measurement, evaluation and competition system is not enough. Data and outcome systems often can be manipulated to give the illusion of quality care. No matter how managed care companies are measured, their tendency to undermine quality and interfere with accessibility continues. Later in Chapter 11, "Patching-up Insurance Driven Health Care," the many reasons why such systems cannot work will be explained.

Can competition save managed care?

When the managed care scheme was invented, it was promoted as a system in which the managed care companies would compete for quality and accessibility. Competition among managed care companies is supposed to counterbalance the dynamics that lead to declines in quality and accessibility. To make competition work for consumers, consumers need real choices over selecting and changing managed care companies, and they do not have this choice.

Employers, not consumers, usually select the insurance or managed care company, and they have a different agenda than consumers. To switch managed care companies, employees must either change jobs or hope that the employer responds to employee requests for a different managed care company. Changing insurance coverage might require changing providers, thus disrupting important provider-patient relationships. Even when consumers individually purchase their own insurance, pre-existing conditions usually are not covered for a period of a year, and sometimes even excluded. Individuals with pre-existing conditions are often much better off "stuck" with a poorly performing managed care company than with a new company that will exclude coverage for their health needs.

It is so impractical for consumers to change to another managed care company that they are, in effect, trapped with their insurance plan. With captive customers, managed care companies may dictate the cost and conditions of service. Managed care companies also dictate to patients which doctors can be seen and what kind of service is authorized. Because consumers have lost their freedom to choose another managed care company, competition does not prevent a decline in quality and accessibility.

The negative effects of managed care are not merely hypothetical; they are something that many consumers have experienced. Patients already have run into the problems in managed care. Indeed, many consumers and providers have stories to tell about how they had to battle to get needed health care. At times it may take a persistent, well-informed, energetic, and assertive patient or patient advocate hours of struggle with a managed care company to obtain needed care.

Can managed care be fixed so that it does not harm the quality of care?

Can managed care be fixed? The answer is yes, but only partially and at a great expense. A regulatory structure can provide some protection for patients. A complex and expensive appeal system, with professional advocates, could represent patients who are not able to fight the battle themselves. A complicated system of quality controls can be established. The problem is, of course, that if regulation is added to control the excesses of managed care, then managed care becomes increasingly more expensive. As it is more expensive, one has to question whether it adds enough value to make it worth the cost. The most expensive health care system in the world becomes even more expensive.

Single Payer Systems

Single payer systems are a monopsony, a close relative of the well-known monopoly. A monopoly occurs when all of the production of goods or services is controlled by one entity. A monopsony occurs when all of the consumers are controlled by one entity. The single owner or operator of the monopsony, by controlling the choices of all consumers, can demand that providers lower their prices. While monopsonies are powerful in cutting costs, they create unhealthy market dynamics. Monopsonies can be just as bad as monopolies. In fact, in recognition of their ability to be harmful to markets, both monopsonies and monopolies are violations of the Sherman Anti-Trust Act.[9] Both take away consumer choices. Once consumer choice is gone, providers have less incentive and innovation suffers. Both are so

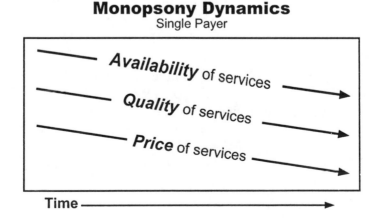

Monopsony Dynamics
Single Payer

Availability of services

Quality of services

Price of services

Time

powerful that they undermine healthy market forces and, consequently, excessively lower quality and undermine the needed availability of goods and services.[10]

The monopsony controls all consumers and can set prices, quality of services, and standards for accessibility. In some ways, government control over consumers is better than managed care because governments are transparent. Managed care has a veil of proprietary secrecy that often hides its cost-cutting policies and practices, whereas governments are open to public review. Voters and elected representatives can improve and correct the system. The government does not need to make a profit on the administration of the system, and administrative costs of government-operated single payer systems are much lower than in managed care.

The critics of a single payer system point out that even though single payer systems are economical, low in administrative expenses, transparent, and monitored by open government, the negative effects of monopsonies endure. Every single payer system in the world partially controls costs by setting up queues, or waiting lists, that delay services. Accessibility and the shortage of providers becomes a problem. Likewise, quality suffers because single payer systems are slow to incorporate innovation.

The other fear of a United States single payer system is based on the country's record of creating an enormous bureaucracy when it does anything. Providers roll their eyes and cringe when they think about government health care systems like the Veteran's Administration, Medicare, and Medicaid. These systems get stifled with bureaucracy. They justifiably fear that a Canadian-style system in the United States would result in a bureaucratic nightmare.

Single payer proponents have two solid arguments in their favor. Such a system would provide universal coverage, and it could alleviate the burden on employers of paying for health care, workers' compensation health care costs, and other health care liability costs. The advantages and disadvantages of the single payer system are further explained in Chapter 12, "Single Payer Compared to Balanced Choice."

The Current Quagmire

Our current health care systems are in a quagmire. Despite the complex multitude of systems, in 2003, 45 million Americans, one out of seven, were uninsured, and the number is rising.[11] One out of four is without insurance for some part of a two-year period.[12] It is difficult to correct problems that are entangled in multiple competing insurance companies and government operated systems. Great efforts to make incremental improvements have resulted in little movement in this quagmire.

This nation does not have a "health care system." Indeed, there are, at the present time, seventeen different health care systems. Many of these contain numerous subsystems. They are poorly integrated.

1. Medicare
2. Medicaid
3. Children's Health Program
4. Native American Health Program
5. CHAMPUS—Program for military personnel and their dependents.
6. Federal Employees Benefits Administration—Program for federal employees.
7. State, county, and city health benefits programs
8. The Veterans Administration
9. Armed Forces Health Programs—Programs for military near military bases
10. Employer purchased employee health insurance
11. Individually purchased health insurance
12. Specialized health services as provided by state, county, or municipal governments
13. Emergency care used by the uninsured
14. Direct payments out-of-pocket by some consumers for some health services
15. Workers' Compensation for health care expenses
16. Automobile Insurance liability for health care expenses
17. Other liability insurance, including malpractice awards, for health care expenses

Almost every system has its own set of rules and requires small, medium, or large administrative and bureaucratic structures to administer and to "police" them. Some of these, such as employer-based health care insurance, have multiple companies offering complex systems that might include

PPOs and HMOs. Such a complex morass of systems has led some to say that it is an oxymoron to talk about the U.S. Health Care System.[13]

This collection of seventeen systems results in the most expensive health care system in the world, costing 147% as much per person than the next most expensive, Switzerland.[14] In terms of quality of care on many measures, the United States lags far behind many countries. Life expectancy and infant mortality statistics place the United States in the bottom quartile of industrialized countries.[15] When treatment outcome for 21 conditions was compared among Australia, Canada, New Zealand, England, and the United Sates, the United States only came out best for only one condition, breast cancer survival.[16]

In these overlapping systems, when a person is covered by two or more insurance policies, instead of patients being reassured by double coverage, they are often abandoned by two systems that fight over who has to pay the bills. When auto insurance or workers' compensation provides coverage, it is not uncommon for patients to need to hire an attorney in order to obtain payments because these companies are so reluctant to pay. A solution to the problems in the health care system must find a way to decrease the inefficiency of the multiple systems and the wasted resources spent in boundary disputes between systems.

Stuck in the quagmire of the current systems policymakers try to initiate incremental change and are afraid of any real movement. There are four choices:

1. Staying in the quagmire of the current systems
2. Moving to more managed care
3. Moving to single payer
4. Moving to a functional market in Balanced Choice

Understanding health care economics makes it possible to look at how the problem might be fixed. In other words, if the problem is in the economics of the system, the solution is to find a way to change the economic system that underlies health care financing. Balanced Choice does just this. The next chapter explains how Balanced Choice solves most of the problems in health care by developing a functional market that restores consumer choice.

Chapter 3—Balanced Choice:
A Functional Market System

Summary: Balanced Choice provides health care security for all, and unlike insurance and single payer systems, it maintains consumer cost consciousness through the use of gap payments. It is a comprehensive health care system with two basic Plans: a Standard Plan that assures universal coverage and an Independent Plan in which consumers and providers have choices that enhance the Standard Plan. Balanced Choice includes a Mandatory Funding Split that assures that the Standard Plan will always have adequate funding for quality care and maintains a balance between the Standard and Independent Plans. These features create a health care security system that has functional market forces, which lower prices, raise quality, and improve accessibility.

How does Balanced Choice avoid the dysfunctional economics of other proposals for funding health care? Why does it work better? Because it has three basic components that create both health care security and functional market forces. First it establishes a Standard Plan that assures universal coverage. Second, in the Independent Plan, a gap payment system establishes a functional market and offers options that enhance the Standard Plan for providers and consumers. And third, a Mandatory Funding Split assures that the Standard Plan does not become substandard and functions to maintain a balance between the Standard Plan and Independent Plan.

A Standard Plan That Assures Universal Coverage

Balanced Choice begins by creating the Standard Plan to assure universal coverage. Regardless of financial status, everyone can receive quality health care in the Standard Plan. In some respects, this Plan is similar to Medicare, a system that provides health care security for millions of beneficiaries. Like Medicare, the Standard Plan provides comprehensive coverage for all necessary health care services at an affordable rate. In fact, Balanced Choice is similar enough to Medicare that the Medicare reimbursement schedule could be used as the starting point for Standard Plan reimbursements.

Although similar to Medicare, it is best to think of the Standard Plan as enhanced Medicare. It includes a substantial pharmacy benefit, good mental health benefits, long-term-care benefits, and a mechanism to assure that reimbursement rates are not set too low to attract quality providers. The Standard Plan requires some copayments and gap payments, but unlike Medicare, Balanced Choice would assume responsibility for these payments for low-income patients or patients with catastrophic health care expenses.

Are there any gap payments in the Standard Plan?

In the current health care systems, patients usually pay a portion of their health care expenses. In the Standard Plan, except in cases of financial hardship, patients would continue to pay a portion of their health care expenses. For medications, imaging and lab expenses, Balanced Choice would make a base payment for each service, and patients would pay the gap between the base payment and the actual charges. Because of gap payments, consumers would be cost conscious. Gap payments are explained in more detail in the description of the Independent Plan.

Are there any copayments in the Standard Plan?

Patients would also be responsible for small copayments for appointments with providers. A large portion of the health care community believes that it is important for patients to take responsibility for their own health care by paying something for each visit. Regardless of whether copayments make a difference in patient responsibility, Balanced Choice believes this viewpoint should be accommodated. In addition, because patients pay a copayment for provider visits in the current system, Balanced Choice strives to continue current sources of funding and require some payment. Gap payments, in this situation, do not make sense because all Standard Plan providers must follow the same reimbursement schedule. Therefore, the required payment is a copayment.

Copayments potentially do create one important problem, however. Even small copayments can be an enormous barrier to low-income patients. To solve this problem, Balanced Choice does not require any copayment from anyone on the Standard Plan for the first two visits each year. Once low-income patients enter the system, they are advised about how to apply for Balanced Choice financial assistance with copayments and gap payments if necessary for their future care.

If everyone is in Balanced Choice, is it a monopsony?

In a monopsony, one entity controls the choices of all consumers. Because, in Balanced Choice, both providers and patients have a choice of using either the Standard Plan or the Independent Plan where fees vary, Balanced Choice is not a monopsony.

The Independent Plan and Gap Payments Restore a Functional Market

In Balanced Choice providers may charge more than the Standard Plan fee schedule by opting for the Independent Plan. With each new patient, providers would choose which Plan would be used. Providers can also transfer Standard Plan patients to the Independent Plan if they give patients a year's prior notification.

In the Independent Plan, patients are charged a gap payment for provider visits. For each type of service Balanced Choice has a fixed base payment. Patients pay the gap between the base payment and the price charged by a provider.

The base payment and gap payment system is quite different from the way insurance-driven health care attempted to provide health care security. Because the treatment of many illnesses became too expensive for all but the wealthy, insurance-driven health care promised to pay most of the cost. It said that if patients first pay a copayment (first dollars), insurance would pay the remainder (last dollars) regardless of how much the health care cost was. With this system, consumers lost cost consciousness. Only the party that pays the remainder (last dollars) cares about a price increase. In Balanced Choice it is reversed, Balanced Choice first makes a base payment (first dollars) and patients pay the gap payment (last dollars).

Not all insurance plans paid last dollars. Some made an attempt to instill cost consciousness by requiring that patients pay 20%, 30%, or 40% of the cost. Theoretically, this should make consumers cost conscious, but it is a diminished cost consciousness. Because insurance is still paying 60%, 70%, or 80%, patients have the same lowered cost consciousness that a consumer might have at a sale in which everything was discounted 60%, 70%, or 80%. For example, if the cost of a service increases $10, and insurance pays 60%, then a patient would only pay $4 for the $10 increase.

31

It is not much wonder why these percentage copayment plans have not had the power necessary to contain inflation in health care.

Balanced Choice, on the other hand, requires that consumers pay 100% of a fee increase. When consumers are paying the full cost difference, they are cost conscious. With cost-conscious consumers, the primary need for managed care is eliminated.

Cost comparison information

Attempts at restoring cost consciousness in consumers have been stymied in the past by the difficulty consumers have in obtaining relevant cost information. When patients and doctors choose a medication in the doctor's office, relative costs of medications are unavailable. Differences between charges for imaging or lab tests are also unavailable. Even when a consumer asks providers, hospitals, imaging services, or labs about costs, they often cannot get the information because charges change depending on the patient's insurance company. Many insurance companies have proprietary pricing arrangements with providers, and these companies only inform consumers of the costs after procedures are completed and after the proprietary price adjustment has been made. Without comparative price information, consumers cannot make cost-conscious decisions.

Balanced Choice includes ways to make cost comparison information available to consumers. Providers can offer so many different services that a complete price list from providers would include too much information. It would be impractical for consumers to collect and compare such lists. In order to make price comparison among providers convenient, Balanced Choice requires that Independent Plan providers base their fees on a percentage of the Standard Plan reimbursement schedule. Thus, one Independent Plan provider might charge 115% of the Standard Plan reimbursement and another might charge 120% of the Standard Plan reimbursement.

By basing provider fees on a percentage of the Standard Plan reimbursement, consumers easily can obtain information about how provider charges compare. Information can be made available about typical gap payments for procedures and for the average long-term treatment of various health conditions, based on the percentage charged by an Independent Plan provider. With this price comparison information, patients could decide if the value of the Independent Plan provider was worth the cost for the individual patient's situation and preferences.

Price information about medication, lab tests, and imaging tests would be handled differently. Each of these providers would be required to publish, quarterly, a list of their maximum price for each service or product. Pharmaceutical companies, labs, and imaging services would be able to sell their products or services below the maximum price; however, they would also be motivated to strive for the lowest possible maximum price because consumers would be using the price lists to make their choices. Specifics about this price comparison are described in more detail in Chapter 7, "A Balanced Choice Pharmacy Plan."

Can patients make wise choices about comparing costs versus benefits?

Some people express concern that if consumers are comparing costs, they will not have the expertise to make wise health care decisions. Of course, consumers rarely have the expertise to make decisions about different medications, labs, and imaging services without expert guidance. This is why Balanced Choice requires that the cost comparison information be so widely published and circulated that it is available in the doctor's office where consumers can receive expert advice. In the case of medications, consumers would be able to choose a less expensive medication only if the provider agreed that it was a proper medication for their health condition.

Balanced Choice Dynamics

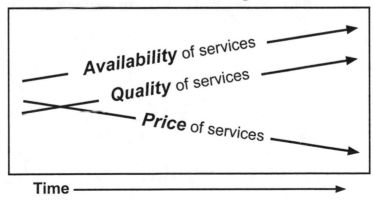

What is the functional market created by Balanced Choice?

Balanced Choice is different than other health care system proposals that claim to be "market-based proposals." Most of the "so-called" market proposals are ways to move money in the health care marketplace, but not ways to establish functional market dynamics that lower prices, raise quality, and improve accessibility.

Balanced Choice features that establish functional market dynamics:

- *Consumers have continuous unbundled choices* of goods and services. HMOs are an example of bundled choices—each HMO bundles together a limited selection of providers, medications, and a set of internal policies that restrict treatment options, and consumers are restricted from easily changing HMOs. In Balanced Choice, there are no bundled choices like enrolling in an HMO. Consumers have the choice of Plan and the ability to change providers or Plans at all times.
- *Consumers have easy access to the information necessary for comparison* of cost, accessibility, and quality. Balanced Choice provides consumers with cost-comparison information whenever needed including when they consult with their providers.
- *A substantial portion of the population is able to afford the choices.* Balanced Choice sets reimbursement rates that assure that nearly half of the patients can afford and will choose the Independent Plan.
- *Providers are allowed to set fees* that the market will support. Balanced Choice sets the floor for provider charges in the Standard Plan, and Independent Plan providers are free to set fees as high as the market will bear.
- *A provider's ability to change Plans is not restricted.* Balanced Choice allows providers to choose which Plan will be in effect for each new patient and to change Plans with adequate notice.
- *The decision makers are consumers,* not third-party entities, such as employers, government, or managed care companies. The interests of other entities are never completely aligned with consumers, and consequently, will always have some negative impact on quality or accessibility.
- *There is an effective cost containment mechanism.* Balanced Choice uses the base payment and gap payment system to contain costs by maintaining cost consciousness in consumers.

Mandatory Funding Split: Keeping the Two Plans Balanced

Two-tiered systems have been rightly criticized because they are vulnerable to having the standard tier gradually starved of funding and deteriorating into substandard care for the poor. Public hospitals, public mental health systems, and recent cuts to Medicaid are examples of how health care systems are under-funded if they are seen as systems only for the poor. Maintaining quality in the Standard Plan depends on a mechanism that protects it from being starved of funds and, consequently, deteriorating.

The necessary protection is created by the Mandatory Funding Split— a requirement that the Balanced Choice board set Standard Plan reimbursements and Independent Plan base payments (the amount Balanced Choice pays to providers) at rates that result in 60% of Balanced Choice funds going to the Standard Plan and 40% going to the Independent Plan (a 60/40 split). To ensure that reimbursement adjustments are gradual and responsive to changing markets, in a manner similar to the Federal Reserve Board, the Balanced Choice Governing Board is required to evaluate and six times a year, make the adjustments needed to maintain the 60/40 split.

Because consumers and providers have choice over whether they use the Standard Plan or the Independent Plan, Balanced Choice must maintain this 60/40 split without coercion. To maintain the 60/40 split, the Balanced Choice Governing Board must use reimbursement policies to entice consumers and providers to select Plans in a manner that results in the 60/40 split.

How do reimbursement policies maintain the 60/40 split?

To understand how the Mandatory Funding Split protects funding for the Standard Plan, it is helpful to first review how the Standard Plan and Independent Plan providers are reimbursed.

- *Standard Plan reimbursement*—If the Standard Plan schedule sets a basic doctor's visit reimbursement at $100, in most cases the patient pays a $10 copayment and Balanced Choice pays the remaining $90 directly to the provider. For each visit, the Standard Plan has $90 credit toward its mandated 60%.
- *Independent Plan reimbursement*—Independent Plan re-imbursement is more complicated. Balanced Choice does not pay

the full Standard Plan fee to the Independent provider. Balanced Choice pays the Independent Plan provider a base payment of a percentage of the Standard Plan fee. In this example, the Independent Plan reimbursement percentage is 85% of the Standard Plan. Thus, Balanced Choice pays the Independent Plan doctor 85% of the $100 Standard Plan fee or $85 as a base payment. If this doctor charges 115% of the Standard Plan fees, the doctor's full fee would be $115. The base amount paid by Balanced Choice is $85 and the patient's gap payment is $30. For each visit, the Independent Plan has $85 credit towards the mandated 40%.

If the system starts to move away from the mandated 60/40 split, the Balanced Choice board can make four adjustments to entice providers and consumers to make choices that restore the 60/40 split.

1. Increase Standard Plan reimbursements to entice more doctors to accept more Standard Plan patients (e.g., raise Standard Plan reimbursements 5%)
2. Decrease Standard Plan reimbursements to entice more doctors to only accept Independent Plan patients (e.g., lower Standard Plan reimbursements 5%)
3. Increase the base payments to Independent Plan providers by increasing the Independent Plan reimbursement percentage, which consequently decreases the gap payment and entices more patients to use the Independent Plan (e.g., increase Independent Plan reimbursement percentage from 85% to 90%)
4. Decrease the base payment to Independent Plan providers by decreasing the Independent Plan Reimbursement Percentage, which consequently increases the gap payment and discourages patients from using the Independent Plan (e.g., decrease Independent Plan reimbursement percentage from 90% to 85%)

Why is the Independent Plan base payment less than 100% of the Standard Plan reimbursement schedule?

In order to contain costs, it is important that the Independent Plan is never reimbursed 100% of the Standard Plan reimbursement. If 100% were covered, it would be too easy for providers to restrict themselves to the Independent Plan. They could do so by charging a slightly higher percentage rate than the Standard Plan (e.g., 102% or 104% of Standard Plan reimbursement). Very few providers would accept only Standard Plan reimbursement, and there would be no way to protect health care quality with so few providers. The Standard Plan could then indeed become substandard care for the poor.

In addition, if 100% transferred, it would encourage inflation. Most consumers would not hesitate to pay small increases, and it is the repetitive small increases in costs that are an important contributor to the escalation of health care costs.

Why is the split 60/40?

More Balanced Choice funds are likely to be spent in the Standard Plan for several reasons. All emergency room care is under the Standard Plan. Patients with catastrophic or chronic illnesses are more likely to use the Standard Plan because these illnesses impact income and raise health care expenses. The split should allow for these increased expenditures through the Standard Plan.

The concept of the split is key to providing the balance that makes the system successful; the exact ratio used to describe the split is illustrative, but fairly accurate. In the later phases of developing Balanced Choice, more detailed analysis and mathematical modeling may suggest that there be a different split.

Is it too complex to set reimbursement amounts for all medical services?

Currently, the Center for Medicaid and Medicare Services (CMS) already sets reimbursement amounts for all medical procedures for Medicare patients. In Balanced Choice, the Balanced Choice Governing Board would assume responsibility for creating this reimbursement schedule and, in many cases, would begin by adopting the Medicare schedule. Where the reimbursement rates have been too low to attract quality providers, the Governing Board could make the necessary increases.

Are the Balanced Choice board's adjustments actually government price controls?

No, they are not price controls. Providers always have the alternative pricing structure of the Independent Plan. In fact, because of the Independent Plan, it is better to think of the reimbursement adjustments as policy decisions that follow the market. For example, jobs in the public sector often have salaries comparable to similar jobs in the private sector, and in this way the public job salaries follow the market. Likewise, if Independent Plan providers earn substantially more income than Standard Plan providers, the Balanced Choice board would be pressured to follow the market and raise Standard Plan reimbursements.

What effect do the Balanced Choice board's adjustments have on inflation?

A mathematically sophisticated reader will be aware that the 60/40 split can be maintained with many combinations of Standard Plan reimbursement schedules and Independent Plan reimbursement percentages. If the Balanced Choice board set both of these too high, it could cause excessive inflation in health care, and if it set them too low, it could cause health care income to fall below the rate of inflation. The Balanced Choice board would be required to set the combination of Standard Plan reimbursement schedule and Independent Plan reimbursement percentage at a point that resulted in overall health care provider incomes increasing at the same rate of inflation as the rest of the economy.

Conclusion

The Standard Plan, gap and base payments, and Mandatory Funding Split are the essential components of Balanced Choice. These three components create a comprehensive health care financing system that provides universal coverage, has healthy market dynamics, and protects the Standard Plan from being underfunded.

Chapter 4—An Outline
for Financing Balanced Choice

Summary: Balanced Choice is financially feasible. By eliminating the high administrative expenses in the United States health care system, Balanced Choice could achieve a substantial savings, some of which would be used to meet the additional costs of the health needs of the uninsured. A large portion of the savings would be set aside to reduce the employers' contributions to health coverage. Balanced Choice proposes that health care funding could be provided by maintaining government and out-of-pocket sources at their present levels and converting both the reduced employers' payments and the current employees' payments for health insurance to a fund dedicated to paying for Balanced Choice health care.

Is Balanced Choice financially feasible? Can Balanced Choice be implemented for less money than is currently spent on health care? If it saves money, what might be done with that money? How might Balanced Choice be financed?

Savings Created by Balanced Choice

The United States already spends enough on health care that it can more than afford a health care system that has high-quality universal coverage. The current hodgepodge of seventeen different systems and a marketplace of competing insurance companies have created the most expensive health care system in the world, costing 47% more than the next most expensive system.[17] The key to financing Balanced Choice is finding a more efficient way to spend the funds that are already there.

Balanced Choice can create this efficiency by decreasing administrative costs. The conglomeration of United States systems has an enormous bureaucracy and administrative structure that siphons funds away from the delivery of health care. Providers and their staffs must spend a large portion of their time fulfilling the diverse bureaucratic requirements of these different systems. Single payer systems have much lower administrative costs. Balanced Choice, because it is a single system, would be just as efficient.

The administrative costs of the U.S. health care systems have been compared with the administrative costs of the Canadian single payer system in a 2003 analysis by Woolhandler and Himmelstein. They found that the administrative costs of the U.S. were 31% and in the Canadian system comparable costs were 16.7%. Although this study may underestimate the savings, it still indicates that by converting to a single payer system, the U.S. could save at least 14.3% of the National Health Expenditures (NHE—an estimate by the Centers for Medicaid and Medicare Studies of the amount that is spent on health care in the United States annually). In terms of the 2004 NHE, the conversion would achieve a savings of $258 billion.[18]

Distribution of Administrative Savings Created by Balanced Choice

Current U.S. health care	Balanced Choice
Administrative expenses $560 billion	Not allocated—$50 billion
	Reduce employers' contributions $100 billion
	Health care for those previously uninsured $108 billion
	Administrative expenses $301 billion

This comparison is based on data from the 2004 NHE.

To be conservative, the $258 billion figure is used here; however, there are good reasons to suspect that the actual current saving would be substantially higher. Woolhandler and Himmelstein found that difference between administrative costs in the United States and Canadian was increasing. Our health care system continues to become more complex. It is very likely that a study conducted today would show that administrative costs have grown even larger, which would mean that the conversion savings would be higher.

It will become a Balanced Choice priority to develop more current and accurate estimations of the full savings that can be achieved by an administratively simpler system. For now, the conservative estimate of $258 billion is sufficient to show that Balanced Choice would generate enough savings to cover the uninsured as well as to reduce the cost of health care in the United States.

Covering the Uninsured

Establishing universal coverage is the first priority for using the savings created by conversion to Balanced Choice. Fortunately, paying for the additional health care costs of the uninsured is not as large an expense as might be imagined. The uninsured already receive substantial health care services.[19] Some of their uncompensated care is subsidized by cost shifting from patients with insurance. In other words, the fees for health care for those with insurance are high enough that they can offset the amount providers lose by treating those who cannot pay. Other times, the uninsured become eligible for public health insurance like Medicaid after they are impoverished by a medical condition. Some of the uninsured pay out of pocket. All of these payments for the health care for the uninsured are already included in calculating the NHE.

Balanced Choice only needs to find additional funding to provide for the uninsured's neglected health care needs. It is estimated that only an additional three to six percent of the NHE would have been needed to fully cover the uninsured in 2001.[20] To be conservative and assure that enough money is available for quality care, Balanced Choice uses the upper end of the range—six percent. With this estimate, $108 billion[21] would have been needed to cover the uninsured in 2004, the most recent year for which data is available. The $258 billion savings created by a conversion to Balanced

Choice can cover this $108 billion and still have $150 billion savings for other parts of the health care system.

Providing Relief to Employers

Providing employers some relief from the high cost of furnishing health care is a priority for Balanced Choice. Currently, the high cost of health insurance is a barrier to hiring new employees, and consequently, it restricts job growth. In the long run, businesses in the United States need to be more able to compete efficiently in the global marketplace. Because American employers have had to carry the burden of health insurance, they have been at a disadvantage when competing with countries whose employers do not have such a major burden. Reducing this load on employers is not just good for employers; it is good for the country.

Balanced Choice proposes lowering employers' current total contribution to health care by at least $100 billion. Their current contribution consists of the employer's contribution to purchasing health care insurance, paying the medical portion of automobile insurance, and paying the medical portion of workers' compensation insurance. In place of this contribution, employers would contribute to a Balanced Choice Health Care Fund by paying a percentage of the employee's wages. This contribution, when calculated for all employers, would collect $100 billion less per year than the employer contribution in the current system.

Employers would achieve additional savings. Their benefits departments would no longer have any responsibility for health care administration. Their employees would no longer lose time learning about health insurance and dealing with the benefits department concerning health care.

In conversion to Balanced Choice, businesses should be promised that they would not have any future tax increases to pay for funding health care. If more funds are needed, the additional funds should come from another source, not businesses. Health care should be a national concern, not an employer's concern.

These changes would not affect all employers in the same way. Those who have been paying for the major costs of health care will likely have a great savings. On the other hand, the Wal-Marts and McDonalds, those who have not been paying for health care, will experience the contributions to the

Balanced Choice Health Care Fund as an additional burden. To ease this adjustment, contributions for these employers would be phased in over a two-year period. This phase-in will likely cause wage expenses to rise at no greater than the rate of inflation.

Where Will the Other Balanced Choice Funds Come From?

As much as possible, Balanced Choice would obtain funds from sources that are already paying for health care in generally the same proportions that they have been paying. In 2004, the states and the federal government paid $824 billion or 45.7% of the National Health Expenditures.[22] This funding would be transferred directly to the Balanced Choice Health Care Fund. Employers would continue to pay a portion, although a smaller one, through the proposed employer's contributions to the Balanced Choice Health Care Fund.

Out-of-pocket expenses, gap payments, and copayments would continue to contribute the same share of the NHE as they do currently. In Balanced Choice, however, the out-of-pocket expenses would be more equitable. In the current system, out-of-pocket medical expenses are often disastrous, causing 54% of the bankruptcies filed.[23] In Balanced Choice, most out-of-pocket expenses would be voluntary for those who choose to use the Independent Plan. If expenses were too burdensome, patients could choose the less expensive Standard Plan, and if they qualified for financial assistance, could have Balanced Choice assume the copayments and gap payments. There should be no more bankruptcies caused by medical expenses. Reductions in bankruptcy help businesses and financial institutions as well, because they do not have to absorb unpaid debt.

Employees would provide most of the funds for the remaining costs. Instead of contributing to the cost of their health insurance and paying for the medical portion of their automobile insurance, employees would make contributions to the Balanced Choice Health Care Fund based on a percentage of their wages.

The overall amount that employees contribute to the Balanced Choice Health Care Fund would not be greater than they are now paying for health insurance and the medical portion of automobile insurance; however it would impact employees differently. Those who presently pay a portion of their wages for health insurance will continue to pay a similar, but probably smaller, amount in the form of an employees' contribution to a Balanced Choice Health Care Fund. Those who have not had insurance will begin paying a portion of their wages to health care. Balanced Choice would smooth out variability in the system in which some employees pay a large portion of their health care, some pay a small portion, and some pay none but are uninsured. In place of the variable system, employees would pay for health care at the same rate, a percent of their income. In return, employees would be assured that they would have consistent health care coverage even if they are unemployed or change employers.

Conclusion

For less money than is currently being spent on health care in the U.S., Balanced Choice can provide health care for everyone. A conservative estimate indicates that $258 billion would be saved by conversion to Balanced Choice. Of this amount, $108 billion is needed to cover the uninsured, $100 billion is designated to provide employers relief from the burden of health care, and $50 billion is undesignated. Funding for Balanced Choice would come from the same general sources that currently pay for health care. What the employees currently pay for health insurance and most of the funds that employers currently pay for health insurance would be transferred to a Balanced Choice fund.

More specific expense and funding estimates are needed. In the next phase of Balanced Choice development, there will need to be a more comprehensive analysis of the savings realized from reducing administrative costs. It is likely that the administrative savings would be substantially greater than the preliminary conservative estimates. Mathematical modeling is needed to estimate how the Standard Plan and Independent Plan can prevent health care costs from excessive inflation.

No health care proposal has the answer for the constantly increasing technology and its associated costs. Expenses are rising also because more health care is available and people are living longer. People value health and want to spend more on health care as medical science has more to offer. It is not reasonable to think that health care should be frozen at some portion of the GDP. The growth in health care expenses will happen regardless of the system that is used for financing health care. With Balanced Choice, though, consumer cost consciousness should slow the growth as well or better than other proposals.

Establishing a health care system without provisions for increased future funding is contrary to common sense and a way to guarantee a system's failure. Without this provision for additional funding, any system, even Balanced Choice, will eventually run out of funds. The final Balanced Choice proposal will have recommendations for how and when the United States might need to consider increasing funding for health care.

Balanced Choice is financially feasible. It is a leap forward in financing health care, can provide more for less, and can contain unnecessary expenses. Balanced Choice can solve health care funding needs for the near future and slow the rate of rising health care costs.

Section III

The Experience
of Balanced Choice

Chapter 5—The Consumer-Friendly Experience in Balanced Choice

Summary: Balanced Choice is easy and straightforward for consumers to understand and use. Everyone is always covered and consumers are presented with one choice at a time. The consumer's experience using Balanced Choice is described in more detail by addressing questions about eligibility, selecting or changing a provider, selecting or changing a Plan, choosing medications, obtaining lab and imaging tests, gap payments, hospitalization, emergency treatment, and long-term care.

For you, the consumer, obtaining health care is easy and straightforward with Balanced Choice. When you see your providers, you would talk about health concerns and recommendations—not about insurance coverage. While you may consider cost in choosing different treatment options, there is never a question about whether necessary treatment is affordable.

Balanced Choice makes purchasing health care much like other consumer purchases. Consumers consider their needs, possible services, possible benefits, potential drawbacks, and the cost. There are often goods or services that vary in quality and cost, but are satisfactory. A discount grocery store and an upscale grocery store both offer nutritious food. Private colleges and public universities can both offer quality education. With Balanced Choice, you have similar choices about how to match your personal needs and preferences with treatment choices and compare the cost of each choice.

In two important ways, however, Balanced Choice is different from other parts of the consumer economy. First, in Balanced Choice you are guaranteed access to necessary health care. You never need to fear that you will not be able to afford treatment for an illness or other health condition. People with incomes insufficient to allow them to make copayments or gap payments can have their payments covered by Balanced Choice. Balanced Choice also covers the copayments and gap payments for people with expensive catastrophic illnesses.

Second, quality care is assured even in the less expensive plan, the Standard Plan. Balanced Choice financial incentives mandate that Standard Plan reimbursements are high enough so that providers willingly choose to treat Standard Plan patients at least half of the time. These financial incentives are also substantial enough so that at least half of consumers will choose to use the Standard Plan, even when many of them could afford the Independent Plan.

Answers to Consumer Questions about Balanced Choice

What would I need to do to be eligible for Balanced Choice?

You need only to contact Balanced Choice to obtain a patient identification number, and then you are eligible for health care. In an urgent situation, you could receive your number immediately. Once the number is obtained, it is good for your lifetime. You never need to do anything else to have health care security.

How would I select a provider?

Good health care is built on the foundation of a trusting personal relationship with a competent provider. In Balanced Choice, this relationship would be exclusively between you and your provider—there would be no hidden contracts with managed care companies, no preauthorizations, no utilization reviewers attempting to restrict care, and no hidden guidelines limiting necessary care. Balanced Choice covers all providers. You could choose which provider to contact by using professional recommendations, personal recommendations and any other information you desire.

You would also have the opportunity to consider the cost of treatment. After selecting possible providers, you would ask one or two cost-related questions. "Are you accepting new Standard Plan patients?" If the answer were yes, you could just make an appointment. That would be the least expensive option, and there would be no need to look further.

If the provider answered that he or she is accepting only Independent Plan patients at this time, then the second question would be, "What is your Independent fee schedule?" All fee schedules would be based on a percentage of the Standard fee schedule. One Independent Plan Provider might charge 110% of the Standard fee schedule, and another might charge 115%. You could also ask for other cost estimates such as the gap payment for an initial meeting. If you thought the fees were acceptable, and that the provider visit was worth the gap payment, you could make an appointment. If you thought the fees were too high, you could continue to look for a provider accepting Standard Plan patients or an Independent Plan provider with lower fees.

What would a Standard Plan doctor visit be like?

A Standard Plan appointment with a provider would focus exclusively on health care, not questions of insurance coverage. The only administrative procedure would be making your copayment. If further treatment were recommended, there would be no need, however, to check to see if it were covered by insurance because Balanced Choice covers all necessary treatment. You and your provider together would consider treatment based on the potential benefits, possible risks, and cost.

What would an Independent Plan doctor visit be like?

Like the Standard Plan, an appointment with a provider would focus exclusively on health care, not questions of insurance coverage. Independent Plan provider visits would usually offer more benefits than the Standard Plan. These benefits might be the provider's excellent reputation, greater experience, or special qualifications. A doctor might offer more immediate appointments or might schedule longer appointments. Instead of making a copayment at the beginning of the visit, in the Independent Plan you would make your gap payment at the end of the visit once the full charges were known. As with the Standard Plan, if further treatment were recommended, there would be no need to check to see if it were covered by insurance. You and your provider would together consider treatment based on the potential benefits, possible risks, and cost.

Would I get stuck with an inadequate provider on the Standard Plan?

Some fear that the Standard Plan would become a haven for inadequate providers while most quality providers would only be available through the Independent Plan. This would no more be true in Balanced Choice than it is in the current managed care systems in which the choice of providers may be limited for those who accept a lower fee. The state licensing boards and professional groups would still regulate quality of providers. You would have a choice of numerous providers in the Standard Plan and could avoid or leave providers whom you found to be undesirable.

Providers have many reasons for accepting Standard Plan patients. They may need to fill a new practice, want the security of knowing that their practices are full, or to have a desire to see patients who cannot afford Independent Plan fees. While not all providers will see Standard Plan patients, there would be a large selection of competent professionals, more than currently is available in most managed care networks.

How could I select low cost medications?

Choosing medications can be complicated, and you would usually want the guidance of your physician. Because not all medications in a category are interchangeable, providers would still need to decide what medications were advisable. To bring price consideration into the medical office, Balanced Choice would give all providers up-to-date and easy-to-use medication gap payment comparison charts. You and your provider would know the anticipated gap payment for various acceptable medications at the time you choose your medications.

Because cost is a concern to you, your provider might say, "I am recommending this type of medication and there are three possibilities. Some patients have more side effects with the least expensive one, but we could try it if you like. If you have side effects, we can choose another one even though it is more expensive." Cost conscious consumers would often try the less expensive medication. Medications would compete on price and value, just as various brands in a grocery store do. Often, you would be able to save money by choosing a less expensive medication. Marketplace competition would lead to reducing the cost of many medications.

If you preferred to have your provider make the choice of medications, you could also save money. Even when your doctor made the decision, he or she could choose the least expensive one appropriate to your needs. This would be quite different than the current system in which providers tend to be aware only when there is a large price difference between medications.

How could I choose low-cost lab and imaging tests?

You would have control over the size of your gap payments for lab and imaging tests. If tests were recommended, you could shop around for lower gap payments, or your provider might be able to give you information about gap payments at local laboratories and imaging centers. If the most convenient locations had higher gap payments, you could choose between convenience and cost.

Lab and imaging are sometimes a matter of discretion. To further control health care costs, you could ask about the importance of recommended tests, and when there is some room for personal discretion, you could consider the cost versus the potential benefits. You would have control over the cost of your care, and your cost-consciousness would keep prices from rising unnecessarily.

What about deductibles?

There would be no deductibles in Balanced Choice. Coverage begins with first visit to a provider. In cases of catastrophic health care expenses, the gap payments may be decreased as expenses rise.

Why should I have to pay any gap payments?

Someone on the health care system needs to watch costs and be concerned about excessive costs. Without gap payments, either the government or managed care would be deciding what is an excessive cost and what treatments are worth the cost. When there are gap payments, consumers and the consumer-provider team are the ones concerned about costs, and the consumer-provider team retains control over health care decisions.

Would copays and gap payments keep me from getting necessary care?

Balanced Choice is a system that eliminates barriers to health care. To encourage early diagnosis and prevention, the first two primary care visits each year in the Standard Plan would have no copay. If you were unable to pay, Balanced Choice would accommodate your situation. Standard Plan providers would inform patients that, if needed, assistance is available. The medical office could give you a simple form requesting Balanced Choice assistance with copays or gap payments.

What about hospital care?

Hospitals would offer both Standard and Independent Plan beds, but the difference between the two plans would not be in the delivery of essential medical services. Before deciding to choose an Independent Plan hospital bed, you could ask about the Independent fee schedule, the anticipated gap payments, and the Independent Plan benefits. Independent Hospital benefits could include a higher staff-to-patient ratio, private rooms, better accommodations for relatives who spend time with you, or other additional benefits.

What about emergency care?

There is often no time to ask about the cost of treatment or to make choices in an emergency. You would always be covered by the Standard Plan for treatment at emergency rooms and trauma centers.

What about long-term care?

Essential long-term medical care is no different than any other medical service in Balanced Choice. Even in the current system, Medicaid pays for most long-term care. In Balanced Choice, you would be expected to pay the residential portion of your care as long as you are able, but the medical portion would be paid on either the Standard Plan or the Independent Plan. Independent Plan long-term care benefits might include a greater staff-to-patient ratio and additional services.

Conclusion

In Balanced Choice, consumers assume their rightful place as cost-conscious decision-makers in health care. This cost consciousness not only lowers the cost of your individual health care, but also creates a market force to lower the cost of health care. By assuming responsibility for cost consciousness, you reap great benefits. You gain the ability to have a patient-provider relationship free from the interference of managed care or the influence of insurance companies. The system is able to save enough money to provide everyone with health care. You gain complete health care financial security.

Chapter 6—The Provider-Friendly Experience in Balanced Choice

Summary: Balanced Choice respects providers as professionals and business people. Balanced Choice is designed to meet their financial needs and contribute to job satisfaction. The Balanced Choice provider experience is described by answering questions about selecting which Plan to use, setting fees, mixing patients from each Plan in a practice, adequacy of reimbursement, limitations on government controls, regional differences in reimbursement, limitations on regulations, limitations on managed care, the authority of providers, payment guarantees, gap payments, and the effect of Balanced Choice on malpractice insurance.

Providers are the heart and soul of the health care system. They supply the services that are valuable in health care. Their professional responsibility is the main safeguard for quality. Balanced Choice addresses provider job satisfaction and interests and respects them both as medical professionals and as business people.

How do the two Plans work for me if I am a provider?

Each time that you accept a new patient you agree with your patient whether payment will be through the Standard Plan or the Independent Plan. You merely need to tell new patients either that you are accepting Standard Plan patients or that you are accepting only Independent Plan patients.

If you accept patients on the Standard Plan, you agree to be paid according to the Standard Plan reimbursement schedule and to collect a small copayment from your patient at the beginning of the appointment. Balanced Choice pays the unpaid portion of the fee. If patients are low income, they may have their copayment paid to you by Balanced Choice.

If you accept patients on the Independent Plan, you tell them your fees in relationship to the Standard Plan fee schedule. For example, you may charge 110% or 115%, or any other percentage of the Standard Plan fees.

Balanced Choice pays a portion of the Standard Plan fee schedule, and you collect the remaining gap payment from your patient.

> Example: If the Standard Plan reimbursement for an office visit is $100, and you charge an Independent Fee of 115%, your fee would be $115. Balanced Choice pays you a set portion of the Standard Plan reimbursement, which in this example is 85% or $85 (85% x $100). The gap between your fee and the Balanced Choice payment is $30 ($115–$85 = $30). You collect the gap payment ($30) from your patient at the end of the appointment and bill Balanced Choice for $85.

This system is somewhat like the current difference between being an in-network provider and an out-of-network provider. Patients now have low copayments for in-network providers but the provider needs to accept a lower reimbursement. Patients pay more to see an out-of-network provider. The difference is that Balanced Choice is more flexible for you than the current system. You can make decisions whether to use the Standard Plan or the Independent Plan one patient at a time, and in your practice, you can have any mixture of Standard Plan and Independent Plan patients that you develop.

Can I switch patients between the two Plans or change Independent Plan fees?

Yes, you can change fees or change patients from one plan to another. There are just a few guidelines.

When you want to lower Independent Plan fees, this is to your patient's advantage, and you may do so at any time. Also, if your patient could not continue to afford Independent Plan fees, and you wanted to continue treating that patient, you could switch that patient to the Standard Plan at any time. Again, this is to your patient's advantage.

If you raise Independent Plan fees, it is not to your patients' advantage, and therefore, you would need to give a three-month notice. If you want to change your patients from the Standard Plan to the Independent Plan, it is also not to your patients' advantage, and in this case you would need to give a one-year notice. During the notification period, your patients may choose to find a more affordable provider.

Why would I treat Standard Plan patients if I can earn more on the Independent Plan?

Filling your practice is easier in the Standard Plan because it is less competitive and many patients will be unable or unwilling to pay the higher gap payments under the Independent Plan. When you are starting your practice or having difficulty filling your practice, you may find it advantageous to take Standard Plan patients. The reimbursements under the Standard Plan will be adequate, or they will be increased. If providers, overall, do not opt to treat Standard Plan patients at least half of the time, as mandated by Balanced Choice, reimbursement rates for Standard Plan procedures will be increased to encourage providers to treat more Standard Plan patients.

Accepting Standard Plan patients is no different than accepting the reduced fees from managed care plans in the current health care systems. Accepting these reduced fees depends on the adequacy of the fees and the advantages of maintaining a full practice.

Why would consumers pay the Independent Plan gap, when they can receive quality care in the Standard Plan for a small copayment?

Consumers value choice. They have demanded that insurance plans have out-of-network coverage because they do not want to have their choices restricted. Many consumers will pay a premium for services from a highly recommended professional, a professional with additional training, a highly experienced professional, or a professional who shows special interest or caring.[24]

Why should I be restricted to charging a percentage of the Standard Plan fee?

Someone in the health care system needs to be cost conscious. If it were not the patient who is cost conscious, then it would be government or managed care that made decisions about cost. Patients, however, need some standard way of comparing prices, because it would be too complicated for consumers to be able to compare a myriad of health care costs for different treatments and procedures. By basing charges on a percentage of the Standard Plan reimbursement schedule, Balanced Choice offers a compromise that gives providers the freedom to set their fees and consumers a way to compare costs.

Would it work for me to have a mix of patients and for patients to have a choice of plans?

As a professional in the current systems, you have experience dealing with multiple payment plans, and therefore, a mix of patients. The difference in Balanced Choice is that there are only two plans, and you set your own fees in one of the plans. You also would not need to keep track of multiple payment schemes; the amount of reimbursement from Balanced Choice for each procedure is as close as your computer.

How do I know that I will receive adequate reimbursement from Balanced Choice?

In Balanced Choice you are able to earn an income that is commensurate with your training, expertise and hard work. Balanced Choice addresses your income needs in both Plans. The Standard Plan is mandated to maintain a high enough fee schedule so that, collectively, providers voluntarily treat Standard Plan patients at least half of the time. You may refuse new Standard Plan patients if you believe that the reimbursement is not satisfactory.

In the Independent Plan, you can raise your fees higher than the Standard Plan. Providers with strong reputations, special training, and greater expertise can be compensated with greater income. The Independent Plan also allows you to charge higher fees if you offer additional benefits that persuade patients to pay the gap fees.

Is Balanced Choice a government-run health care system?

Providers have justifiably resisted the idea of a government-operated health care system. This is not an abstract ideological position, but one that is based on experience with government systems. Medicare has a history of unilaterally determining reimbursement rates that do not adequately reimburse some areas of health care. In the current system, you can refuse Medicare patients because there are other sources of income. If there were only one system, it is natural to be concerned about having your profession crippled by misguided government policies. At times Medicare has also made heavy-handed threats of prosecution for fraud and huge fines when providers have made errors in following bureaucratic procedures.[25] The Veterans Administration is known for bureaucratic inefficiency.

Balanced Choice is not this kind of government program. It protects providers from these abuses because it allows patients and providers to make choices. Providers are not locked into accepting the fee schedule and can use the Independent Plan if the Standard Plan fees are insufficient. Balanced Choice would be required to distinguish between bureaucratic errors and fraudulent billing, and it would be prohibited from the heavy-handed threats of criminal prosecution that were used by Medicare. It is not a health care delivery organization; it is a payment system for independent providers of health care services.

What about regional differences in reimbursement?

Balanced Choice responds to regional marketplaces. Balanced Choice is required to set reimbursements so that it maintains the balance between Standard Plan and Independent Plan both nationally and regionally. If reimbursement were too low in a regional marketplace, providers would insist on using only the Independent Plan in order to obtain adequate reimbursements. With too many providers refusing Standard Plan patients, Balanced Choice would not achieve the requirement that, collectively, the reimbursements need to result in over half of all patients being treated in the Standard Plan. The system would be out of balance. To restore the balance, reimbursements in such a region would need to be raised. Likewise, if rural areas could not attract both Standard and Independent Plan providers, reimbursements in these areas would need to be raised to attract enough providers so that both Independent and Standard Plan providers are available.

Isn't it better for providers to have a market system rather than a controlled system?

A market system is usually better than a controlled system. Unfortunately, in the current system that has been called a free market, it is really only the insurance companies and their customers, the employers, that enjoy a free market. Using their power, insurance companies have regulated and controlled consumers and providers as severely or worse than a government-run system could. Balanced Choice allows consumers and providers most of the benefits of a free market while both establishing the financial support that consumers need in order to afford health care and creating a safety net so that no one needs to go without health care for financial reasons.

Will Balanced Choice regulate my practice?

Balanced Choice is not a system for regulating health care; it is a payment system. The regulation of health care will be independent of Balanced Choice. State governments and professional organizations would remain responsible for the licensing and regulation of health care.

Is there any managed care in Balanced Choice?

Balanced Choice is designed to minimize the regulation of health care. The primary justification for managed care has been controlling costs. In Balanced Choice, because consumers are responsible for gap payments, consumer cost-consciousness would restrain costs.

Balanced Choice, however, is not a rigid ideological system. It is designed to work. In order to be practical, Balanced Choice recognizes that there are some areas of health care that can benefit from a limited form of managed care. A good example is the excessive use of inpatient psychiatric treatment in the 1980s. Because insurance was paying the bills, for-profit psychiatric hospitals developed expensive inpatient treatment programs that were unnecessary and at times even contraindicated. To prevent these abuses, when there is clear evidence of wasteful treatment, Balanced Choice may require treatment reviews, which could be conducted within the following guidelines:

- The review process must demonstrate that the review is beneficial and that the cost and inconvenience are justifiable.
- The review process would need to be completely transparent. Guidelines, how they are established, and how they are implemented would be subject to open discussion. There would be no more secret managed care guidelines, anonymous reviews, or covert negotiations with utilization reviewers.
- Utilization reviewers would not be able to overrule treatment decisions without examining the patient, thoroughly reviewing the history, and fully consulting with the treatment provider.

Would Balanced Choice interfere with treatment decisions?

As providers, you are the best people to make treatment decisions, and Balanced Choice maintains your independence and central role in making health care decisions. You have the direct involvement with patients, and in Balanced Choice, you have the personal and professional responsibility for the quality of health care. Neither third party utilization reviewers nor bureaucratic guidelines can produce better decisions than yours. Balanced Choice supports your independent judgment and professional authority.

Balanced Choice allows treatment decisions to be made by the provider-patient team. It is not a system of managed care. In Balanced Choice, consumers are cost conscious. It is the provider's role to guide patients in deciding when treatment is necessary, when it is optional, and how patients can safely reduce expenses.

Can I be assured my patients can pay for necessary treatment?

Balanced Choice provides universal coverage, and your patients will never need to forego necessary treatment due to financial constraints. Balanced Choice will pay you for the treatment that you provide, and your patients will be able to obtain assistance from Balanced Choice if they are unable to pay their copayments or gap payments. In the first visit each year, your patients will be notified that they can obtain assistance from Balanced Choice if they are unable to pay their portion. All providers would have paperwork and instructions that could be given to your patients to start the process of applying for assistance. You will never need to turn a patient away due to the lack of coverage or financial resources.

If there is only one system, what happens if payments are delayed?

Balanced Choice would require that all claims be paid within ten working days of when they are received. There is no reason why an organization whose only responsibility is the financing of health care cannot respond within ten days. The current practice of insurance companies waiting 30 or 60 days to respond is merely to help their cash flow and increase profits that come from investing their reserve funds. It is not related to the complexity of paying claims.

How can consumers be expected to pay a gap for expensive services, hospitalization, or surgery?

To meet the needs of all providers, there will be some difference in the Standard and Independent Plans reimbursement rates for different services and providers. Primary care providers, cardiologists, and neurosurgeons have different issues. Likewise hospitals and long-term care facilities have their special concerns. Balanced Choice will develop reimbursement rates that are acceptable to all specialties and facilities as Balanced Choice continues to evolve. The reimbursement schedules will be guided by the mandate that providers will choose to see Standard Plan patients at least half of the time and gap payments will be reasonable enough that patients will choose to pay Independent Plan providers nearly half the time.

Will Balanced Choice help with malpractice insurance?

Balanced Choice will lower malpractice awards, and to some extent, the frequency of malpractice claims. Because Balanced Choice provides birth-to-death health care coverage, malpractice claims will no longer include compensation for future health care coverage. This will lower the size of claims. In addition, some malpractice claims are filed because patients or their parents feel obligated to obtain an award in order to cover future health care costs. For example, if a child has a disabling condition, loving parents often feel that they must do whatever necessary to obtain funds for their child's future health care. Sometimes this means a malpractice lawsuit. If health care coverage is guaranteed, these obligatory lawsuits will be eliminated, and consequently, there will be fewer lawsuits.

Conclusion

Balanced Choice is designed to be good for professionals, consumers, and employers. It respects the expertise, professionalism, and income needs of providers while still offering increased benefits for consumers and employers. It restores the importance of the provider-patient relationship. Because providers are no longer spending hours serving the needs of insurance managed care companies, it will lead to greater job satisfaction.

Chapter 7—A Balanced Choice Pharmacy Plan

Summary: The Balanced Choice Pharmacy Plan establishes functional market dynamics that lower prices, raise quality, and improve accessibility. Pharmaceuticals have not competed on the basis of price, which has resulted in continuous increases in the price of established medications. Balanced Choice restores functional market dynamics through three features. It makes a price comparison list available to providers and patients, assures that consumers have an expert provider available when they make decisions about medications, and encourages consumers to be cost conscious by requiring a gap payment. The Pharmacy Plan offers promise for greatly lowering the cost of medications without government price controls. In addition, the Pharmacy Plan can be implemented to repair the unpopular and flawed Medicare Part D program.

The Balanced Choice Pharmacy Plan demonstrates how Balanced Choice creates a functional market and lowers the cost of medications. It is an example of how providers and consumers can conveniently use price information when making treatment decisions. In addition, the Pharmacy Plan is one aspect of Balanced Choice that can be implemented independently of the entire Balanced Choice package. This offers the possibility of a stepwise transition to Balanced Choice. By becoming a replacement for the unpopular Medicare Plan D, Balanced Choice can lower costs, make the plan consumer-friendly, and greatly improve coverage.

Pharmaceutical Market Dynamics

The current pharmaceutical market is dysfunctional.

In functional markets, when there are competitors, prices are supposed to decline. The opposite is happening with pharmaceuticals. The cost of medications that have been on the market for years, usually medications that have competitors, are rising as much as 360% of the rate of inflation.[26] If prices had been decreasing as a result of market competition, this would have offset some of the increases in medication costs for new products and increased medication use in the general population.

How is it that the market does not work to lower costs of medications that have competitors? The pharmaceutical market effectively prevents providers and consumers from being fully cost conscious in several ways. First, price information is extremely difficult to obtain. Providers and patients do not have price information available in the doctors' offices where the medications are chosen. Second, because most insurance companies charge a flat copayment for prescriptions, cost differences between medications do not matter to most patients. And third, cost increases are so gradual that they are not visible to providers or patients. For example, 50 of the most prescribed drugs for seniors had an average of an annual 4.9% price increases in the five-year period ending in January 2003.[27] As a result of the obscurity of price information, consumers and providers can only be aware of large price differences or the difference between generic and brand name medications.

The health insurance industry has made some ineffective attempts to simulate price competition. Many managed care companies created drug formularies—books that rate the cost of medications in a manner similar to the star systems used by movie reviewers and by creating barriers to obtaining medications thought to be too expensive. Unfortunately, formularies function more like annoying bureaucracy than a market force. Other managed care companies intercede when prescriptions are taken to the pharmacy and pharmacist benefit managers attempt to persuade providers to change the prescription to less expensive medications. The use of pharmacist benefit managers is time-consuming and highly abrasive to patients and providers. The current fad is to have three-tiered systems with a different copayment for each tier. The low copayment tier is for generic drugs; the middle copayment tier is for medications that are favored by the managed care company due to price, negotiated special deals, or rebates; and the high copayment tier is for drugs considered expensive. Tiers save money for managed care companies that may have negotiated a special deal or rebate from a pharmaceutical company for including a medication on the second tier, but these negotiations do not change the price of medication for the rest of Americans.

These attempts to simulate price competition do not discourage pharmaceutical companies from their practice of small, but frequent price increases. These small increases are not large enough to affect a medication's star rating in a formulary or move it from one tier to another. Even if an insurance company does restrain a pharmaceutical company from small increases by contractual arrangements, the pharmaceutical company still can raise prices for other customers.

Traditionally, pharmaceutical companies have argued that the price increases are essential to pay the costs of research and development. However, this is not where they allocate the majority of their revenues. The top seven pharmaceutical companies in the United States spend an average of 14% of their revenue on research and development but allocate 18% to profits and 32% to marketing, advertising, and administration.[28]

Balanced Choice corrects the market dysfunctions.

Balanced Choice has three features that make the pharmaceutical market functional. First, Balanced Choice creates price lists by requiring that drug manufacturers publish the maximum price for their medications. The published price is used by Balanced Choice to create a cost-comparison chart for the typical dose at a typical pharmacy—the expected retail price list. Medications can be listed easily in groups with similar medications so that costs can be compared at a glance, just as is done with various brands of food in the supermarket. Even small increases or decreases in the price of a medication would show up on the list, and thus there would be normal functional market pressure to keep prices as low as possible. The list allows doctors and patients to make price comparisons, and it also shows patients the amount of the anticipated gap payment they will need to pay for each medication. As with suggested retail prices of many other products, consumers can often obtain additional savings depending on where they shop.

Second, Balanced Choice assures that consumers have an expert medical advisor available when making complex medical decisions. It has been argued that consumers are not knowledgeable enough to make health care decisions. While it is true that consumers usually need a knowledgeable advisor in order to make wise health care decisions, this is no different than numerous other areas where consumers use expert advisors. When making legal decisions, consumers consult attorneys, and when making tax decisions, consumers consult accountants. In health care, consumers use their physicians as their expert medical advisors.

In the Balanced Choice Pharmacy Plan, consumers are not left alone to compare the costs and benefits of various medications. Just as always, the doctor makes the decision about which medications can be prescribed. The only difference is that price information is handy, and consumers can ask their doctors to consider price when choosing among similar medications.

Third, Balanced Choice maintains consumer cost consciousness by having patients make a *gap payment*. Balanced choice pays a base amount for each category of medicines, and patients pay the full *gap* between the base amount and the actual charge for a specific medication. The following example shows how gap payments work.

Simplified Example of Balanced Choice Expected Retail Price List
(This is a list of three medications in the same category)

Medication	Retail price	Balanced Choice pays pharmacy this base amount for medications in this category	Patient's gap payment
Medication A	$45	$40	$5
Medication B	60	40	20
Medication C	65	40	25

In this example, Balanced Choice pays the same base payment of $40 for all medications in the category regardless of the cost of the specific medication. Patients pay the gap between the base amount and the actual cost. If the doctor and patient select Medication A, which costs $45/month, the patient pays a gap of $5/month. If the doctor and patient select the higher priced Medication B or Medication C, the patient pays a gap of $20/month or $25/month respectively.

Example of how Balanced Choice works in the doctor's office— a fictional dialog.

> Dr. Goodheart: Considering your history of heart problems and high blood pressure, I would like to start you on a beta-blocker.
>
> Mrs. Beewell: Okay, but my finances are tight so I would like you to consider cost while choosing a medication.
>
> Dr. Goodheart: Gladly, I know that cost matters. I have in my hand, here, this month's Balanced Choice expected retail price list. There are five beta-blockers, but only three that I would consider prescribing for you. Now on this chart, the lowest priced one would have a gap payment of $30 per month, but more patients report side

effects with that one. The next lowest priced one would have a gap
payment of $39 per month and fewer people report side effects.

Mrs. Beewell: Why don't I try the $30-per-month one for a couple of
weeks, and if I get side effects, I will try another?

Dr. Goodheart: Good idea. We have a plan. I will see you in two weeks
to see how well the medication is working.

(As it turned out, Mrs. Beewell found a discount pharmacy that
lowered her gap payment to $21 per month and the less expensive
medication proved to be just right for her. Overall, Mrs. Beewell
found her annual gap payments were lower than her combined
copayment and deductible costs on the health insurance she had
before the Balanced Choice Pharmacy Plan.)

There is tremendous power that will come from the cost-conscious patients
using the Balanced Choice expected retail price lists to select medication.
Once providers are sensitized to price, they will probably consider price
differences even with low-income patients who have the full cost of their
medication paid by Balanced Choice. The market will change from the
current situation, in which drug companies hardly ever face real price
competition, to one where there are few places to hide from real price
competition. The result should be a functional market in which there is a
steady decline in the price of established medications.

It is true that one medication cannot always be replaced by another in the
same category, and therefore no two drugs are equal competitors. Two
medications in the same category may be equally effective for only some
patients. This is no different than most other parts of the free market
system. Competitors are usually not offering identical products, and they
still compete on price.

Will price competition work for medications? Of course it will; it does
in every other sector of a functional market. Other countries have tried
versions of the Balanced Choice plan called "reference pricing." Most
notably, Germany has had reference pricing on some medications since
1989. In the time period from 1989–2001, the *price index for reference-
priced medications decreased 30%* while the price index for medications
not reference priced rose 25%.[29] Although some other cost-control measures
during this time period made it difficult to evaluate the precise effect of
reference pricing, it shows that there is great potential for price competition
to reverse the rising cost of medications in the United States. It would

be a great accomplishment if, in the United States, the Balanced Choice Pharmacy Plan would take 30% or more out of the bloated prices that have developed in the years without price competition.

When price competition begins to work, it will restrain medication costs without requiring government cost controls that might stifle the invention of new drugs. After all, it is well established that price competition is a traditional component of functional market systems and is known to stimulate innovation and new products. Pharmaceutical companies, just as other industries that cope with price competition, will be able to make healthy profits.

The Balanced Choice plan also saves money because it eliminates most of the administrative costs that occur in both managed care entities and government bureaucracies. The Balanced Choice plan requires minimal administration to distribute price lists and to make the base payments directly to pharmacies.

There is another bonus that comes from the Balanced Choice plan. Critics have blamed expensive direct-to-consumer advertising for pushing up the cost of medications. The pharmaceutical industry defends itself by saying it is only educating consumers about the possibility of improving their health care. If the Balanced Choice plan is implemented, when Mrs. Beewell sees Dr. Goodheart and inquires about the medication she heard about on TV, he might say, "Yes, you have that condition, and because I know you care about cost, let's see how much each of the different medications for that condition cost." When advertising expenses push up the cost of the medication, the advertiser may lose the sale in the doctor's office if its medication is not competitively priced.

The difficulties in implementing the Balanced Choice Pharmacy Plan should not be exaggerated. Other countries that have used this system have had a single payer system, and consequently, consumers were very reluctant to pay significant gap payments.[30] In the United States, on the other hand, consumers are accustomed to paying significant amounts for medications. Gap payments could be designed so that overall, they are no more costly than most consumers are already paying. Categories of medications are already established in the *Physician's Desk Reference* and would only need slight alterations. Moreover, even though individual dosage will vary, the expected retail price list does not need to show an individual's exact gap payment; it only needs to show comparative prices.

The Balanced Choice plan can be designed to pay any desired portion of the overall pharmacy costs—60%, 70% or more, as long as the gap payments are affordable for the vast majority of patients. Furthermore, an essential Balanced Choice concept is that no one should forego a necessary health care service due to lack of financial support. The design could increase the size of the base payment as medication costs rose toward the catastrophic level, and low-income patients would have their gap payment completely subsidized by Balanced Choice.

Using Balanced Choice To Replace Medicare Part D

In order for Balanced Choice to establish a functional market for medications, it needs to have a large enough portion of the entire market to cause pharmaceuticals to compete on price. Establishing such a large portion is possible by converting the Medicare pharmacy benefit to a Balanced Choice Pharmacy Plan. Seniors account for 42% of the expenditures on medications in the United States[31]. In addition to Medicare patients, if there were an expected retail price list available to physicians, the 45 million uninsured, as well as the uncounted millions who have insurance but no pharmacy benefits, would use this list when choosing medications and add their market power to Medicare patients. Once cost-conscious consumers sensitize providers to price, they often consider price differences even when the patient is not paying the bill. With this kind of market power, the cost of medications could be lowered.

The Medicare Part D program needs to be changed. It has been widely criticized for placing the interests of insurance and pharmaceutical companies above the interests of Medicare recipients. Instead of directly paying for medications, the Medicare Part D subsidizes insurance companies which compete to provide complicated prescriptions plans. Because Medicare subsidizes insurance companies without obtaining the lowest possible prices for medications, it is a program that is more expensive than necessary.[32]

Choosing a Medicare Part D plan has been a mind-boggling task. There are an average of 15 of these plans in each state[33] and as many as 67 different insurance plans in some places.[34] Each plan has different premiums, deductibles, copayments, gaps in coverage, medications in their formularies, pharmacy networks, and areas of geographic coverage. As a result of the complexity, beneficiaries and their advisors have been overwhelmed by the near impossibility of determining which plans are best. Even after a plan is selected, when prescribed medications change, it changes which plan is advantageous. As a result of the complexity, many beneficiaries will not enroll, which leaves them uninsured for medications.

Medicare also has major gaps in coverage that result in its beneficiaries being underinsured. Some medications are unavailable on any plan, and many medications and pharmacies are unavailable on each individual plan. A financial gap results in high out-of-pocket expenses for many beneficiaries.[35] For example, patients whose medication costs $5,100 per year will still pay $4,020.[36] It is no wonder that twice as many seniors view Medicare Part D unfavorably as view it favorably.[37]

Until now, the major argument against reforms in the Medicare Plan D program is that alternative proposals have all focused on the government negotiating or setting the price of medications. Such price negotiations are so similar to price controls that these proposals have not been able to overcome economic and political concerns. Balanced Choice is an option that lowers the cost of medications, allows the market to determine price, and is administratively much less complex than subsidizing scores of confusing insurance plans.

Conclusion

The Balanced Choice Pharmacy Plan establishes a functional market for medications. It allows consumers and providers choice of medication, lowers the cost of medications for everyone, and accomplishes all this without government controls over prices. Price competition has been proven to work in other parts of the free market system. It has the added possible benefit of being used to repair the Medicare Plan D program.

Section IV

More Balanced Choice Features

Chapter 8—Science, Education, and Consumer Advocacy

Summary: The evidence-based medicine movement is well established and influential. It calls for health care providers to base their treatment recommendations on scientific evidence. It offers consumers the potential benefits of more effective and efficient treatment, but also has possible risks because it may regulate health care in a manner that restricts treatment choices, makes health care unnecessarily bureaucratic, or results in abuse of the "evidence-based" label. To protect consumers, Balanced Choice establishes some principles for the evidence-based designation. To encourage the beneficial use of evidence-based medicine and the application of appropriate scientific advances, Balanced Choice proposes an energetic patient education program. The Consumer Health Advocacy Organization, which is based on the model of Consumer's Union and its publication, Consumer's Reports, would enable consumers to exert market pressure for treatment based on up-to-date scientific evidence. Balanced Choice is open to using treatment guidelines but only if they are generally accepted to be beneficial. The Balanced Choice approach to evidence-based medicine would give consumers important information about the cost-benefit of various treatments. Through the Consumer Health Advocacy Organization, there would be funds to research specific health concerns that might be overlooked by funding sources that do not advocate for consumers.

Consumer advocates, health care educators, health care regulators, and many health care professionals are calling for increased reliance on evidence-based medicine—a movement that requires providers to use treatments that scientific evidence has shown to be the most effective and to discontinue treatments that scientific evidence has shown to be ineffective, inefficient, or wasteful. Evidence-based medicine supporters cite many examples showing that providers often are not aware of the current scientific evidence and/or do not follow recommendations based on scientific evidence. The supporters argue that not only would health care be improved, but it would also be less expensive if providers were held accountable for following the recommendations of evidence-based medicine.

Evidence-Based Medicine—The Good, the Bad, and the Ugly

The good

Science is the foundation of health care. It continually improves the effectiveness and efficiency of treatment. There are examples, unfortunately, of how the provider community has been reluctant to incorporate scientific evidence especially when it negatively impacts their income or traditional practice. One of the most dramatic historical examples is the common tonsillectomy operation that continued decades after research indicated that routine surgery was not supported by research evidence.[38] Many studies indicate that providers have been slow to respond to current science, and the result is that patients receive less effective or wasteful treatment.

On the other hand, there are many examples of how providers do follow recommendations based on the latest scientific evidence. Doctors tell their patients what the latest evidence says about when to treat high blood pressure with medication, when cholesterol-lowering medication is needed, and how often mammograms are recommended. In other areas, such as the advisability of using heart scans as an early warning for coronary artery disease, the evidence and recommendations are still being debated.

Evidence-based medicine is reassuring to patients and consumer advocates. To the extent that many providers recommend ineffective or out-dated treatment that is not based on scientific evidence, consumers would be much better off if providers were required to recommend only evidence-based treatments.

Evidence-based medicine also seems like a boon to employers and others who pay for health care. Money spent on ineffective treatments is wasteful. By requiring providers to use only the most effective evidence-based medical treatments, the quality of health care could be improved while decreasing costs. Indeed, in some cases the advocates of evidence-based medicine are able to cut costs while improving treatment.

The bad and the ugly

Many respectable groups support the evidence-based movement. Indeed, there is a call for greater accountability in health care, education, and public policy. What could be wrong with a movement to base health care services on science? The problems do not come from science, but from the entities that have the power to interpret the science and assign the "evidence-based" label.

Scientific evidence is complicated and requires well-reasoned scientific analysis. Often scientists disagree. Who should decide what treatments receive the "evidence-based" label? Should it be managed care that decides which treatments are "evidence-based" and which are not? Managed care places heavy emphasis on its own financial interests and creates its so-called "scientific guidelines" behind the veil of proprietary secrecy. Can these secret guidelines really improve health care? Actually, many conditions are effectively treated by medications that were only scientifically tested and approved for a different medical condition, a common practice called "prescribing off-label." Would evidence-based medicine prohibit patients from receiving beneficial off-label prescriptions? Would the creation of evidence-based treatment guidelines result in the inflexibility that is common in HMOs?

A precise description of how the "evidence-based" label can be determined is difficult because there are different kinds of scientific evidence and frequently scientists disagree about what conclusions can be made from the data. Some conditions have a generally accepted best treatment or cure, but many conditions are not curable. When a clear-cut cure is available, physicians tend to provide it, but for the many conditions that do not have a clear-cut cure, there is controversy about how to interpret evidence about the best treatments. Well-reasoned scientific analysis of research usually does not yield clear cookbook answers, but results in complex recommendations that require providers to use their judgment.

Usually evidence-based medicine is not just about using science and accountability; it is also a call for guidelines that end up restricting providers. Such guidelines can make the practice of medicine rigid and bureaucratic. Who should prepare the guidelines? The interpretation of science, like most things, is influenced by politics, power, and money. Scientific advances can increase costs as well as lower costs. Should either the government or managed care companies be allowed to make evidence-based guidelines? Can the guidelines allow for individual patient needs? Will guidelines result in providers spending endless hours in learning how to negotiate managed care mazes in order to offer their patients the best treatment? Great care should be taken in deciding what treatments deserve the label "evidence-based," and in considering the implications of requiring the use of guidelines.

Evidence-Based Medicine and Protecting Consumers

Consumers and payers need a system that responds to the latest scientific advances, offers the most effective and efficient treatments, and encourages professionals to be accountable. Consumers need protection from the attempt to use the "evidence-based" label to restrict or ration good care. Consumers also need to know that their providers can use professional judgment and respond to their individual needs. To balance the benefits and risks in evidence-based medicine, Balanced Choice would establish the following principles for guideline development.

1. Guidelines should only be used when there is a general scientific consensus, and should not be used when there is a significant controversy.
2. The development of scientific evidence-based guidelines should always include full disclosure and transparency. The secretly prepared, proprietary guidelines of managed care do not belong in health care. The content of guidelines, who prepared the guidelines, what scientific evidence was considered, and how cost was considered, all need to be disclosed along with the guidelines. If guidelines are open to scrutiny from the public, professionals, and scientists, the wisdom and value of the guidelines can be openly discussed like all science should be. With full disclosure, consumers would be protected from the "evidence-based" label being applied to guidelines that might be promoted by the self-interest of those who prepared the guidelines.
3. Guidelines should enhance appropriate medical care, not create a bureaucratic maze. Managed care guidelines often require providers to spend hours learning how to negotiate managed care bureaucracies and divert time away from patient care.
4. A guideline system should not undermine the good professional judgment of providers. Providers examine patients and know their history and personality. Patients deserve to have the person who best knows their medical needs working jointly with them to make treatment decisions.

5. Guidelines should not be so rigid that they prevent useful treatments merely because there is not yet a solid body of scientific evidence. Some of the most useful advances in treating bipolar illness, depression, and some schizophrenia have come from the off-label prescribing of medications that have only been scientifically proven to be effective for seizures. A rigid adherence to evidence-based medicine would have prevented this advance and the improved treatment of many other conditions.
6. Guidelines should not prevent patients from making their own decisions after weighing the potential benefits of recommended treatments against the side effects and possible risks. Individual preferences matter, and many patients have personal reasons for choosing one treatment over another.

How Does Balanced Choice Promote Evidence-Based Medicine?

Using energetic education programs, Balanced Choice encourages providers to be current with recent advances and evidence-based medicine. It is open to using prescriptive guidelines when there is a clear consensus of the scientific and professional community.

The Internet

The Internet is changing health care. Consumers have increasing access to health care information and current scientific thinking though various websites. Many proactive consumers bring information from the Internet to their providers and expect their providers to be able to respond to questions about the latest scientific finding. Information and consumer pressure can have a significant impact on the practice of medicine. When even a few patients ask for a response to recommendations or suggestions gleaned from the Internet, a provider's awareness is raised. Once awareness is raised, most conscientious providers strive to evaluate new ideas and information, and as a result, will consider changing their practices.[39] The desire to respond to informed consumers is a powerful incentive for providers to keep current with the latest advances. Moreover, because Balanced Choice eliminates managed care and the hours of time that providers waste negotiating the managed care mazes, providers would have more time to keep current with the rapid advances in medicine.

Consumer Health Advocacy Organization

To enhance the power of consumers in the health care marketplace, Balanced Choice proposes establishing the Consumer Health Advocacy Organization (CHAO). The CHAO is inspired by the success of Consumers Union and it publication, *Consumers Reports*. This organization and publication has shown that a pro-consumer organization can be an effective force in shaping the market by independently evaluating products and services from the consumer's point of view. While the number of people who subscribe to *Consumers Reports* is small, its product ratings make a huge difference in which products are successful and in using marketplace forces to improve quality.

Balanced Choice would provide seed money for the CHAO, which would grow as it sold subscriptions to its publication, which might be called something like *Consumer Health Care Reports.*[40] The CHAO would employ scientists and medical providers to evaluate health care products and services from the consumer perspective. Eventually, the majority of CHAO's income would come from subscriptions. The subscription membership would elect its board of directors, thus assuring that it remained independent.

The CHAO would have several roles.

- It would serve as an independent and constructive critic of Balanced Choice.
- It would provide consumers with information that they need to make health care choices, including both the current thinking in evidence-based medicine and cost-benefit information.
- It would control monies for research so that it could evaluate consumer questions that might not be a priority for provider-funded research, government-funded research, or Balanced Choice–funded research. Such research might include studies in wellness, the use of vitamins, the benefits of alternative care, consumer-focused cost-benefit studies, and the quality-of-life issues resulting from various treatments.

Through the CHAO, the provider's voice and the health care industry's voice would be balanced by an independent consumer-oriented voice in the public discourse of the best use of evidence-based medicine. As a consumer-driven organization CHAO would assure that subjective and life-quality factors, such as side effects, convenience, and personal preferences, were considered in its evaluation of health care recommendations.

Professional organization guidelines

Professional organizations create their own guidelines as scientific evidence becomes clear, and these guidelines become the standard of practice. They also create their own credentialing standards. These guidelines and standards are essential components in the operation of a health care system and would continue in Balanced Choice.

A marketplace for scientific guidelines

Can privately written and evidence-based guidelines fit with Balanced Choice if there is no managed care mechanism? Yes, if there is a real need for guidelines, but *at this point it is not clear that such guidelines could be written or that they are necessary.* Clear guidelines are available for only a few conditions, and these guidelines are often already implemented. Other conditions are so complex that the guidelines are also complex and lengthy, and as a result, providers still need to use their professional judgment in how to implement them.

If guidelines could be developed that would significantly improve patient care, a marketplace solution may be possible without resorting to managed care. Private enterprise or medical schools could prepare guidelines to which individual providers could subscribe. Perhaps centers of medical excellence like Harvard, John Hopkins and the Mayo Clinic could author such guidelines and sell these to providers. By advertising that they subscribe to a certain set of guidelines, providers could assure patients that they keep current with the latest advances in evidence-based medicine.

The success of such a market-based system would depend on the quality of the guidelines. Providers would not purchase these guidelines unless they were provider-friendly, useful, and not overly restrictive. The guidelines would need to offer recommendations that really did create more effective and efficient treatment in order for consumers to prefer that providers were subscribers. In addition, the guideline organizations could offer on-line credentialing, which providers could use to verify that they were current with the latest scientific advances.

Consumers would need to know if the guidelines made a significant difference in their health care. The CHAO could rate the value of various guidelines according to which ones had the most beneficial results for consumers. Other independent consumer advocates and organizations such as the American Heart Association also could rate guidelines.

With marketplace pressure to use guidelines, providers would want to obtain a subscription that kept them up to date on the advances of science in order to attract patients. Because consumers would have a version of the guidelines as well, providers would need to be conversant with consumers who raised guideline questions. Thus, without coercion or rigid government regulation, a marketplace system could encourage providers to be current with evidence-based medicine.

Reimbursement Guidelines

In general, the benefits of science are incorporated in Balanced Choice through the marketplace, thereby avoiding rigid regulation. Balanced Choice emphasizes minimizing regulation, using market forces whenever possible, and improving health care through consumer market pressure. In any system, there are times when regulation may be necessary and advantageous. Balanced Choice is flexible enough to manage care or create regulation when it is clearly necessary.

Market pressure may not be powerful enough to eliminate unnecessary treatment, particularly when it is highly profitable. If there were overwhelming evidence and a near consensus of scientist, consumer, and professional groups that a treatment was ineffective, Balanced Choice could exclude it from payment. At times, in areas of health care prone to overuse, Balanced Choice might establish criteria for appropriate treatments.

Additional research funding

Because Balanced Choice has major responsibility for all health care payments, it is positioned to benefit from any cost reductions. Balanced Choice could use some of its funds to research ways to decrease the cost of care without decreasing quality.

Currently, there is little incentive for research that decreases expenses. For example, there is much research on when to start anti-depressant medication because this creates a profit, but little research on when to stop the medication. Although insurance companies might have an interest in cost reduction, there is little competitive advantage to conducting research that would benefit everyone, including a company's competitors.

The possibility of reducing costs through research has great potential. Balanced Choice could fund research through medical schools on such topics as how the cost of various surgical procedures could be reduced, when medications could be reduced or discontinued, and when the frequency of provider visits could be decreased. Such cost-reducing research is rare in the current insurance-driven health care systems. This cost-reduction research would counterbalance the profit-driven research that seeks out more ways to provide treatment and consequently increases costs.

Conclusion

Increasing the influence of evidence-based medicine is vital to an effective and efficient health care system. Balanced Choice offers ways to incorporate the advances of science with less regulation than traditional government systems and with a transparency that is unavailable in the proprietary world of managed care. It would promote science-based consumer advocacy through the Consumer Health Advocacy Organization and its publication, *Consumer Health Advocacy Reports*. Wherever possible, education and market forces would be used instead of regulation.

Money, power, and politics can affect the use of the "evidence-based" label. Balanced Choice addresses the potential negative consequences of the evidence-based movement by establishing principles for guidelines. All guideline development in Balanced Choice would take place in sunlight without any secret proprietary guideline development. These criteria would also assure consumers that their individual needs and preferences could be met, that their providers could use their own judgment, and that guidelines would not make health care unnecessarily rigid or bureaucratic.

In addition, Balanced Choice incorporates guidelines from professional groups, allows for marketplace guidelines, and has reimbursement guidelines. It energetically promotes evidence-based medicine without intrusive managed care or rigid guidelines.

Balanced Choice is also in a position to fund research. It could directly fund research regarding ways to reduce the cost of health care, and through the Consumer Health Advocacy Organization, it would provide funds for health care research from the consumer's perspective.

Chapter 9—More Features and Innovation

Summary: Balanced Choice offers additional innovations and features that augment the major benefits of universal coverage, functional economic dynamics, and freedom of choice. Balanced Choice has an incentive to develop both short-term and long-term prevention programs. It can improve health care for underserved communities including rural areas, low-income neighborhoods, and ethnic communities. As a comprehensive system, Balanced Choice would provide long-term care. Malpractice awards and malpractice insurance premiums would be reduced because health care is guaranteed. Fraud control could be enhanced because consumers are able to monitor their own health care claims. Balanced Choice provides consolidated information on public health issues and health care trends. As a flexible system, it is open to a broad array of cost-containment strategies.

With Balanced choice, the needs and desires of consumers and providers can be balanced economically in one system. In addition, Balanced Choice offers associated innovations and benefits.

Real Prevention Services

Managed care is a system that has claimed to promote prevention. Indeed, it has instituted some prevention programs such as screening for high-blood pressure and paying for mammograms for women over fifty. These programs are showcases for prevention services. Having a showcase is good for marketing, but it is different from actually emphasizing prevention services in all areas. Current health care systems, including managed care, have little motivation to provide long-term preventive services. Consumers regularly churn through insurance companies and insurance companies are bought and sold, so that few consumers are long-term members in any one insurance plan. Many, if not most, of the patients who benefit from long-term prevention programs end up enrolled in a different insurance company when the monetary savings of a long-term prevention program are realized. As a result, prevention programs are shortsighted. They tend to be more influenced by the quarterly needs for stockholder profits than the long-term health needs of patients.

In Balanced Choice, on the other hand, the system is responsible for birth-to-death health care, on a no-fault basis, for everyone. In such a system, prevention becomes more important because the system will capture the financial savings created by prevention programs. Therefore, it would be fiscally responsible to dedicate a portion of the budget to prevention education and services, and to release a portion of the funds for research in prevention.

Mental Health and Educational Prevention Services

Mental health and counseling services are a clear example of the difference that an emphasis on prevention can make. Seven out of ten of the actual causes of mortality are related to personal behavior.[41] By changing behavior related to stress, diet, exercise, smoking, substance abuse, high-risk activities, and use of safety equipment such as helmets, there is a great potential to reduce health care costs. Research has shown that mental health treatment can result in so much reduction in future medical costs that the savings pays for the mental health services.[42] This is a well-known phenomenon called the medical cost offset. However, it often takes four to five years of medical cost offset for the health care system to recover the cost of the mental health services.[43] In today's system, the short-sighted managed care industry has not encouraged prevention through mental health services, but on the contrary, it has dramatically cut funding for mental health services.[44]

Prevention programs that reduce health care costs would be advantageous to the Balanced Choice system. Because everyone is in the same risk pool, the Balanced Choice system would realize the savings created by quality mental health services and by other effective prevention services.

Disease Management Programs

As a system that is responsible for funding all health care, Balanced Choice has an incentive to promote disease management programs. Often patients with chronic or severe illnesses have their treatment fragmented among so many specialists that there is poor coordination of treatment. In addition, these patients can greatly improve their response to treatment and minimize their disability if they are educated about the management of their illness.

To fill these needs, disease management programs have been developed. These programs assure that all potentially helpful services have been offered, treatment is coordinated, and patients have the knowledge to do the best job of managing their illnesses.

In the long run, these disease management programs would save money by reducing visits to doctors and would also improve the outcome for patients. Balanced Choice could fund disease management either through the traditional provider network or through specialists in disease management. For example, in the traditional provider network, a family practice nurse could be paid to offer a class in the management of high blood pressure; or a disease management specialist could help a diabetic patient coordinate treatment, evaluate diet, improve exercise, monitor blood sugar, manage insulin, and maintain necessary doctor visits.

Incentives for Underserved Communities

Balanced Choice is a flexible proposal that uses financial incentives to meet the needs of Americans. If the regular incentives resulted in too many providers in wealthy communities and too few in rural locations, low-income areas, or ethnic neighborhoods, reimbursement bonuses could be given to providers who locate in the underserved communities.

Long-Term Care

In the current system, insurance does not cover the catastrophic expenses of long-term nursing home care. Many people are forced to spend their entire life savings before Medicaid contributes to their care. A health care security system needs to provide security from birth to death. Balanced Choice would cover the medical part of nursing home care and expect residents or other programs to pay the residential costs. Nursing home expenses would be covered in on both the Standard Plan and the Independent Plan.

Malpractice Claims Would Be Reduced

Rising malpractice insurance costs not only increase the cost of health care, but also have driven many dedicated providers out of practice. This is a serious problem in health care. However, eliminating or drastically limiting protections the legal system provides to consumers is a step in the wrong direction. Fortunately, an associated benefit of Balanced Choice is the reduction in the number of malpractice lawsuits and the size of the awards.

There are multiple factors that contribute to the current use of malpractice lawsuits. For the most part, people do not want to sue anyone. It is an unpleasant and emotionally draining experience. Yet, people who do sue, particularly for malpractice, often believe that they must try to obtain some money to pay for future health care expenses. If a child has medical complications at birth, responsible parents often feel an obligation to litigate for money to provide health care security for their children for the rest of their lives.

Balanced Choice eliminates people's concern about future health care expenses. Because Balanced Choice provides health care security from birth to death, patients and parents do not need to worry about how to pay for future medical bills. They do not need to worry about exclusions for pre-existing conditions or being rejected or cut off by an insurance plan. Many people who previously felt a need to collect money for future health care expenses would not pursue lawsuits, particularly when the merits of the lawsuit were somewhat questionable.

If someone did pursue a malpractice lawsuit, it would not include requests for compensation for future medical expenses because Balanced Choice would cover these expenses. The only damages that would be included in malpractice claims would be punitive, pain and suffering, and loss of income. When the size of claims is lowered, the cost of malpractice insurance is lowered. Moreover, the lowered size of the claim also lowers the motivation on the part of patients and attorneys to sue.

Thus, without any regulation or restriction on consumer protections, the upshot of Balanced Choice would be a decline in the cost of malpractice insurance, a reduction in the size of awards, and a decrease in the incidence of lawsuits. When patients are harmed by medical care and choose not to file malpractice claims, they are still assured that their future medical expenses will be covered.

Controlling Fraud and Billing Errors

A major problem in health care is over-billing and billing for services that were not delivered. This costs billions of dollars annually, and in response, government agencies have used heavy-handed police tactics to scrutinize providers. It is the worst of both worlds, too much policing and too much fraud.

It is not surprising that fraud is so prevalent in a third-party system where consumers are taken out of the loop. Providers arrange payment with a third party, either the government or an insurance company, and the patient is told to sit passively on the sideline and make the copayment. Medical bills and insurance bills are usually too complicated for patients to read. Patient input is considered an additional burden on providers and insurers. Often patients are given an itemized statement that is not written clearly enough for them to determine if it is accurate. This system is a sharp contrast to ordinary expenditures in the marketplace where consumers often are vigilant about making sure they are not over-charged.

Balanced Choice has a common sense solution for these billing errors and fraudulent charges. Every time Balanced Choice makes a payment for services, it would send the patient a statement describing the charges and payments in consumer-friendly language. If patients find what they believe is an over-charge, the patient would simply contact the provider and discuss the possible error. The key innovation is that consumers would receive a refund of a portion of the overcharge and the provider would return the remainder of the overcharge to Balanced Choice. The refund given to the vigilant consumer is an incentive for cost consciousness that would be available in both the Standard and Independent Plans. Balanced Choice would receive a simple document stating that a patient discovered a billing error. Then to complete the loop, Balanced Choice would notify the patient that the provider had corrected the overcharge.

In Balanced Choice, health care would become like other areas of the economy, such as grocery stores or auto repair shops, where identifying billing errors would result in refunds. After all, it is the consumer who is in the best position to know what services were rendered. Errors are corrected without regulatory or police action. Moreover, Balanced Choice can be assured that there are millions of cost-conscious consumers keeping health care payments accurate. Police actions would be restricted to situations of complex fraud and systematic over-billing.

Cost Containment in Balanced Choice

Balanced Choice is not an ideologically based system, but a practical system. A practical system uses what works. Balanced Choice does not emphasize the use of market forces because of an ideological preference for the market. It prefers market forces because they work so well in so many situations and regulation often works poorly. However, in spite of the general benefits of the market and disadvantages of regulation, there are situations in which market forces alone do not solve problems. In these situations, it is practical and necessary to use other tools. As a responsive and flexible system, Balanced Choice can step outside the market system when it makes good sense.

Regulation does have its drawbacks. Managed care can be criticized for offering a 25-cent regulatory solution for a 5-cent problem. Balanced Choice proposes reversing this phenomenon to guard against excessive regulation. Whenever there is a 25-cent problem, Balanced Choice will endeavor to find a 5-cent or cheaper solution. Why not more than a 5-cent solution? There are unanticipated complications to regulatory solutions so the less complexity and regulation the better. The following list describes some of the cost containment features that fit with the five-cent solution rule.

Some services may need additional control mechanisms

Containing hospital expenses is important to the viability of a health care system. One possible strategy is paying hospitals established rates for the treatment of certain diagnoses based on a group average for the cost of treating those diagnoses. These payments are called payments for Diagnostic Related Groups (DRGs). In this type of funding, a hospital receives a set payment for each patient admitted for each diagnostic group. These arrangements encourage efficient use of resources and early discharge when it is appropriate, and they also allow for some patients to have extended stays when necessary. It is a practice that is already in use in many situations.

Under the current system, there is concern that DRG reimbursements can be set too low and undermine necessary care. The key is that reimbursement amounts must be set so that they are adequate and sufficient for providers to offer quality care. Balanced Choice can assure that reimbursements are not set too low because the hospital and patients have the option of the Independent Plan. Hospitals might opt out of the Standard Plan for a specific type of admission if reimbursement rates were too low. For example, a hospital might choose to open a Standard Plan oncology unit, but have only an Independent Plan maternity unit. If the low DRG reimbursements resulted in too few patients being accepted on the Standard Plan, to maintain the Mandatory Funding Split (see Chapter 3, Balanced Choice: A Functional Market System), a resource adjustment would be necessary to raise the DRG reimbursement.

Some services may require a responsible utilization review

The occasional need for a responsible peer review is best demonstrated by the overuse of psychiatric inpatient treatment in the 1980s.[45] As revealed in a national scandal, private psychiatric hospitals often recruited patients for inpatient treatment when the expensive inpatient services may not have been necessary. These patients were treated as inpatients as long as their insurance coverage lasted. As soon as the insurance was exhausted, it was declared that the patient had achieved maximum hospital benefit, and the patient was discharged. While managed care was able to stop this, it created problems associated with under-treatment rather than over-treatment. Managed care has set up such stringent barriers to inpatient treatment that patients are routinely hospitalized for only a few days. Even in cases where inpatient treatment is clearly indicated for necessary safety and stabilization—the legitimate reasons for inpatient treatment—hospital stays are frequently denied and patients are often discharged prematurely. Psychiatrists are reluctant to expose these poor practices on a case-by-case basis because if a patient is prematurely discharged, it is the psychiatrist who is most likely to be sued for malpractice.

If the Standard Plan paid for all requested inpatient psychiatric treatment, it could again be overused. On the other hand, having profit-motivated managed care companies restrict hospitalizations is also unacceptable. Because such large sums of money are at stake in psychiatric hospitalization, it is possible for Balanced Choice to pay for independent second opinions about the need for hospitalization. These second opinions would not be conducted by a phone utilization review that is based on five minutes of information, but the reviewers could actually meet the patient, communicate with the provider, and review the record. These independent reviewers would have the authority to set or negotiate hospitalization goals and limits. Such a thoughtful review could be the metaphorical 5-cent solution that saves 25 cents while still assuring that patients who need inpatient treatment for safety and stabilization are able to receive it.

Some patients may benefit from case management

If treatment is uncoordinated, some patients who see multiple doctors may use unnecessary medical treatment to address psychological needs. These patients have been identified as people who consume unnecessary amounts of medical care and, actually, do not get their real needs met. Managed care has promoted itself by claiming that it saves money by providing case management, but it case-manages everyone, even those who do not need it. There is no reason that these complicated patients could not be referred to professional case managers who were paid for their case-management services. In Balanced Choice, patients who need case managers could have them, and case management would not be wasted on those who can best coordinate their own care.

Copayments will be used

Some patient advocates have argued that copayments do not instill cost consciousness for most people because they are like an inexpensive admission ticket. In addition, they argue that copayments are an enormous barrier for low-income patients. Others argue, alternatively, that absolutely free services are overused, and they present some examples to back up this point of view.

Balanced Choice takes a compromise position. The first two annual visits to a primary care provider or emergency room are free of copayment to encourage low-income patients to enter the system when they need medical care. Low-income patients or those with catastrophic illnesses could apply to Balanced Choice for financial assistance for subsequent care so that Balanced Choice would pay the copayments for them. In all other situations, after the initial two medical appointments, Standard Plan patients would make copayments. Independent Plan patients would always make gap payments unless they were treated in emergency rooms.

Balanced Choice Is a Method for Funding Health Care, Not a Method for Regulating It

Attempts to regulate health care often become bureaucratic disasters. In general, as bureaucracies get larger, whether government or private, they become more cumbersome, inefficient, rigid, and unresponsive. For this reason, Balanced Choice is primarily a method for the financing, not the regulation, of health care. Whenever possible, regulation will remain with the state and local governments and with professional groups.

Balanced Choice Would Provide Public Data About Health Care Trends and Epidemiology

In the current system, collecting data on epidemiology and health care trends is enormously difficult. The data is fragmented because of the multiple payers, and because information from insurance companies is proprietary and thus not available to the public. In Balanced Choice, because it is a public system, personally non-identifiable data would be available to researchers, public health officials, and health care economists. This data could be used to detect the possible overuse and under use of services, to contribute to epidemiological studies, and to identify regional trends.

Conclusion

The associated features of Balanced Choice augment its major benefits. Balanced Choice can institute long-term prevention services, improve health care in underserved communities, provide long-term care, reduce the size and frequency of malpractice claims, and control fraud and billing errors. As a flexible system it is open to reasonable cost-containment measures. It accomplishes all of this while remaining a system for financing health care, not a regulatory system. In addition, it can provide valuable health care utilization data that can be used to improve health care delivery.

Section V

Traveling From Here to the Cure

Chapter 10–Health Care Insurance Is Obsolete

Summary: The health insurance industry is an obstacle to health care reform. In order for meaningful health care reform to occur, the problems with the health insurance industry need to be recognized and confronted. Insurance caused the cost-escalation in health care and created the noxious managed care industry. It has financial incentives to shun the seriously ill patients, makes cost comparisons unwieldy, does not have incentives for good service, and inhibits consumer choices. The inherent dysfunctions in the insurance-driven health care system cannot be fixed in an economical or effective manner. Overall, health care insurance does not add enough value to justify its cost. Since Balanced Choice can overcome the problems in the insurance-driven health care system while costing less money, Balanced Choice can render health care insurance obsolete. Proposals are offered for retraining the health care insurance industry personnel.

The health care insurance industry is the elephant in the room where health care reform needs to take place. Many of the problems in health care financing are a result of funding health care through insurance companies. The health care system cannot be cured unless the problems in the health insurance industry are recognized and confronted.

The health insurance industry is the sixth largest lobby in the country.[46] Perhaps because of the industry's power, too many people avoid facing the inherent weaknesses of health care insurance. When Clinton, as a popular President of the United States, tried to reform health care, the insurance industry ran the infamous "Harry and Louise" commercials that killed the Clinton proposal with ridicule within a few weeks. Never mind that Clinton's proposal was a flawed proposal with many other enemies. Having the insurance industry for an enemy was considered the deciding factor. Ever since, politicians and health care advocacy groups have acted as if they are afraid to anger the insurance lobby or as if they are resigned to being in a powerless position.

The question, though, is not whether it is easy to face the insurance lobby. The questions are, what are the real problems and how can they be fixed? Although historically health insurance served a purpose in striving for health care security, it is now becoming obsolete. Health care insurance has fundamental inherent problems that cannot be effectively or efficiently corrected.

Cost-Escalation and Managed Care Are the Result of Insurance-Driven Health Care

Chapter 2, "Making Sense of Health Care Economics," explains how health care insurance undermines consumer cost-consciousness and, consequently, has caused the price of health care to escalate. In an attempt to control cost escalation, the managed care industry was invented. Although managed care has partially controlled medical costs, it has increased administrative costs greatly and harmed the quality and the accessibility of treatment, not to mention aggravating most people who deal with it. Because Balanced Choice does not cause cost escalation and because consumers retain cost-consciousness, there is little need for the expensive and administratively cumbersome managed care system.

Insurance Has Incentives to Shun Seriously Ill Patients

In healthy markets, if people make a better product, they prosper. They attract new customers who want that product, and they make a profit from each customer. In insurance, the incentives are to shun the seriously ill customers, the ones who need insurance the most. A better product, an insurance policy that offers better coverage, can lead to increased losses. This happens because not every customer results in a profit. Healthy people provide the insurance company a profit, while people with expensive illnesses cause a loss instead of a financial gain. If an insurance company offers better products for covering serious illnesses, it attracts people with serious illnesses and high medical expenses. Insurance has invented a term for this phenomenon. It is called adverse selection.

To deal with adverse selection, insurance companies have tried to control who can purchase each insurance product so that few seriously ill patients can enroll. Companies attempt to insure only healthy people who will not need much medical care and attempt *to avoid people who are likely to get sick*.

One way to avoid excessive adverse selection is to insure large groups in which there are mostly healthy people, like groups of employees. In these large groups, people with serious illnesses cannot enroll merely because they want insurance, so the insurance company is protected from adverse selection.

The insurance industry is most vigilant about avoiding people with illnesses when it sells individual plans. If a person has any serious illness, the cost of treatment will exceed the money the individual paid to buy the typical insurance policy. No insurance company wants to sell an insurance policy for $3,000 to a person with $6,000 of medical expense. Therefore, individual policies usually have extensive screening or underwriting examinations that are used to identify people with high medical needs. If the applicant is accepted and covered, individual policies often exclude coverage for a patient's preexisting conditions.

Once people have a serious illness, no insurance company wants to cover them. In Colorado, they are called "the uninsurable" and there is a basic-health-care insurance policy that they are allowed to buy. The cost is high enough, however, that many cannot afford it, especially those who have had their income reduced by a serious illness.

The idea that people who are likely to get sick should pay more for their insurance does not make sense in a health care *security* system. Is illness a failure to be responsible? Sometimes behavior leads to illness, but not always. Asking people who are ill to spend more for insurance is not spreading risk—it is avoiding risk. Moreover, the idea of trying to avoid people who are ill is bound to leave some people out—the uninsured and the uninsurable.

Insurance companies will always avoid insuring people with serious illnesses. It would be fiscally irresponsible to insure them. Quite simply, profits increase more by avoiding enrolling people with illness than by spreading the financial risk of illness over all people who want to enroll.

To entice insurance companies to insure the ill, there have been proposals to have the government subsidize the insurance of people with specific illnesses so that they can then buy insurance. Does it make sense to subsidize insurance so that they do not need to do their job of spreading financial risk? What is the value of insurance then? Such a system would become one in which insurance companies' success depends on obtaining the most lucrative government subsidies.

Balanced Choice, on the other hand, covers everyone. Because everyone is covered by one system, adverse selection does not occur. Balanced Choice does not waste money developing systems to avoid adverse selection. For less money, it does the job that insurance cannot do; it spreads the financial risk of treating illness and injury over all members of society. It creates health care security.

Insurance Makes Cost Comparison Unwieldy

Balanced Choice can rely on consumers being cost conscious because it makes cost comparison information easily available. Balanced Choice standardizes the cost of health care. Standardizing how to compare costs is important in all areas of the economy. In grocery stores, unit cost (e. g. cost per pound or ounce) is usually the appropriate way to compare the costs of various foods. In Balanced Choice, the pharmacy price list shows the cost of the standard dose of medications and the amount of gap payments required. An Independent Plan provider's fees are a percentage of the Standard Plan fee so one provider can be compared with another. Balanced Choice develops appropriate ways to compare costs.

Insurance companies do not have the same option to standardize costs. Standardization requires that there is one standard pricing system. Different insurance companies, however, negotiate different fee schedules with providers. Providers often work for many insurance companies. Negotiated fee schedules can change at any time. Providers could not keep accurate gap payment information readily available for consumers in such a system. Such a system would have so much information that consumers would find it unwieldy to track cost comparison information, and their cost consciousness would be undermined.

Insurance has been trying to restore cost consciousness in consumers. Nevertheless, whatever cost sharing or incentive system insurance develops, it is not as direct as having consumers make the gap payment. Balanced Choice, on the other hand, is effective in maintaining consumer cost consciousness and using price comparisons to control health care costs.

Prepayment plans give poor service

Today's health insurance is not just a way of spreading the financial risk of treating serious illness. It has become a way to prepay for health care. A problem with prepayment plans is that marketing promotions tend to exaggerate the policy's benefits. The financial incentive of the insurance company is to minimize the money returned to consumers. It is like buying a warranty. It looks good when it is purchased, but trying to cash in on the warranty can be filled with hassles and restrictions.

Dealing with insurance companies involves numerous hassles. Phone contact with the company requires negotiating a lengthy telephone tree and spending time on hold listening to recordings stating, "Your call is important to us." Accessing information on web sites can be equally frustrating and ineffective.

The rate of errors in processing claims is impressive. It is difficult to imagine that insurance companies could have so many errors unless they had an incentive to mismanage claims. They do. I call this profitable incompetence. Every dollar not paid out to beneficiaries because of incompetence is a dollar that can go to profit the insurance company.

Aside from incompetence, insurance companies have volumes of proprietary rules and procedures that are intended to limit the amount they pay. Insurance policies and policy manuals are too difficult for most consumers to understand. In fact, I have a Ph.D. and am an expert in insurance, and I cannot tell what an insurance company will do by reading their promotional material, policies, and policy manuals. In practice, there are too many ways that the devilish details can restrict payment.

In any prepayment system there will always be a financial incentive for profitable incompetence or fine-print restrictions on payments. To counterbalance these incentives, it will take even more extensive regulation of the managed care industry than we have today. This regulation will be expensive, cumbersome, and, still, there will be cracks in the regulatory system. Once an insurance company has the money, the financial incentive will be to find ways to keep from returning it to consumers. Consumers and providers who deal with insurance have the experience to know this is true.

Balanced Choice does not have hidden proprietary rules. As a public system, information is transparent and the details of the benefits are available. The rules would be available over the Internet and in hard copy. Independent publishers could write manuals clarifying how to understand what is covered and what is not. There would be no surprises hidden in the fine print of individual policies. As a public system, the incentive is for proper administration, not profitable incompetence. Advocacy groups, the media, elected officials, the Consumer Health Advocacy Organization, and ordinary citizens could expose polices and practices that resulted in mismanagement or other problems.

Patients do not have real choice in selecting health insurance

In a functional market, consumers need to have the option of changing policies when they are dissatisfied; however, this is not the case with health care insurance. If the insurance company does not perform as promised or desired, there is often little a consumer can do to change insurance plans.

When the insurance policy is through an employer, the employee must often change jobs to change insurance. A few companies allow annual choices of different insurance plans, but within the year an employee is stuck. If the company has only one policy, employees need to wait until the company receives so many complaints that it will go through the long and difficult process of finding a new insurance policy and educating all employees about the change. In the end, the new plan is likely to perform as badly as the old plan.

Individuals who have serious illnesses or injuries are most likely to experience problems with insurance, and they also have the most difficulty changing plans. Because of adverse selection, a new company would want to exclude covering the illness because it was preexisting. This exclusion is sometimes for one year and is sometimes permanent. The people who most need health care are the most trapped by the insurance system. What incentive does an insurance company have to make sure that its captive customers receive the best service? The incentive is actually the opposite; it is to the advantage of the insurance company to get rid of patients with multiple claims rather than provide the expensive treatment coverage.

Some people believe that the solution is to get into a good policy when healthy and keep the policy so they have coverage if illness strikes. Unfortunately, the future is hard to predict. Today's good insurance company may run into financial problems or change management at any time. When people believe that they discovered an insurance company that is really above average in performance, experience warns that the situation many change in a few of years. Often, these high-performing companies have a change in management that results in more restrictive payment policies. The financial incentives are powerful and continuously operate to restrict payments.

In Balanced Choice, both consumers and providers always have the choice to switch plans. This choice keeps Balanced Choice responsive to the market and to the experiences of consumers. In contrast, insurance companies must be responsive to their stockholders.

Insurance Does Not Have a True Incentive for Prevention

Managed care has promoted itself as the type of health care that promotes prevention of health problems. This is only true in the most limited sense. Managed care has some high profile ways to emphasize prevention. These showcase services such as mammograms, screenings, and vaccinations have been used to give the illusion of a total philosophy of prevention. The reality is that the financial incentives work against prevention.

Managed care has claimed that prevention actually saves them money, and therefore, it has a financial incentive for prevention. This was the mantra of Kaiser in its early years. It was based on the belief that Kaiser would be responsible for its members for their lifetime, so Kaiser would be interested in reducing the life-long costs of providing health care. The current reality is that consumers often change employers and employers often change insurance companies. If a prevention effort does not reap financial rewards within four or five years, there is no incentive—another company would receive the financial benefits of illness prevention.

This lack of incentive for prevention services is apparent even in Kaiser Permanente, a leader in promoting prevention services. Mental health services have been shown to have tremendous value in preventing disability, decreasing unnecessary visits to medical services, decreasing the need for hospitalization, and in preventing the need for future mental health and physical health services.[47] Mental health treatment's value prevention of physical health problems outweighs its cost. Yet Kaiser has limited mental health services because it requires its staff to maintain such high caseloads that they must limit patients for a few sessions.[48] Meaningful outpatient psychotherapy is almost impossible to receive in their program. If Kaiser had an incentive to pursue the extended benefits of prevention, it is doubtful that they would put so little value on mental health services.

Balanced Choice has an incentive for both short-term and long-term prevention. Because everyone is in the system from birth to death, the system will receive the financial benefits of all prevention services, without the concern that patients could switch to a different insurance plan.

The Enormous Insurance Bureaucracy Does Not Add Value

The real question in a market is whether a product or service adds enough value to justify the cost. The insurance-driven health care system has created, by far, the most expensive health care system in the world. It is also far from the best. Where is the value?

Although some argue that insurance adds some value, is it enough value to justify the time and money costs of administrative expense, indirect provider expense, frustration, consumer time, and employer time? If it does not add enough value to justify the cost and there is a better system, insurance is obsolete.

Can There Be a Mix of Insurance and Balanced Choice?

What if there were a mix of health insurance and Balanced Choice? For example, what about Balanced Choice replacing government programs and providing health insurance for the uninsured, while employers continue to provide insurance? Such a system would avoid confronting the health insurance industry.

It would not work. A double system would undermine many of the benefits of Balanced Choice. It would change Balanced Choice from a health care security system to another insurance company. Balanced Choice would lose its ability to reduce costs. Employers would continue to carry the major burden of health care expenses. The system would not achieve any savings, and the most expensive health care system in the world would become even more expensive.

It does not fix the problems in health care financing to keep insurance along with Balanced Choice. Balanced Choice works because it replaces the hodgepodge of systems with one system. *Balanced Choice is not just another insurance company. It is a national health care security system.*

Can There Be Gap Insurance in Balanced Choice?

In the short-term, gap insurance may seem appealing to those who want the best health care without any out-of-pocket expense. It may also appeal to providers who imagine that it will allow them to charge whatever they wish without discussing costs with consumers. However, to maintain consumer cost consciousness, gap payments need to come from the consumer, not a third party. If there were gap payment insurance, the Independent Plan prices could escalate beyond what consumers could afford without insurance. It would restore insurance-driven cost escalation. This defeats the purpose of making the Independent Plan affordable, and undermines the market forces that come from consumers comparing cost versus value.

Whoever pays the piper calls the tune. If a third party, an insurance company, is paying for the gap, all of the dysfunctional health insurance dynamics would be restored. Gap insurers would divide the risk pool and seek out healthy beneficiaries while avoiding people with illnesses. The size of gap payments would be determined by insurers, not patients, and providers would again need to negotiate with insurance companies. Patients would be trapped once they became ill because no other insurance company would want an ill beneficiary. Insurance companies would have an incentive to avoid gap payments and develop complex procedures and regulations regarding payment. Managed care might be imposed to control cost escalation.

Balanced Choice makes health insurance obsolete only by completely replacing it. This is an either-or choice, either the health insurance mess or Balanced Choice.

Is Any Health Insurance Possible with Balanced Choice?

There is a possible form of insurance that could be purchased by consumers who want additional security if they become ill. It could be designed in a similar manner to disability or life insurance. If a consumer were diagnosed with a serious illness, the consumer could be paid either a monthly stipend during the illness or a lump sum payment as in life insurance. This money could be used at the consumer's discretion for any expenses including loss of income, gap payments, or any other purchase. The consumer would be in charge of how this money is spent. This kind of insurance could be offered with a Balance Choice system because it would not undermine cost consciousness.

Another type of insurance could pay for non-covered services. This might include experimental treatments or non-traditional treatments. This type of insurance would not undermine Balanced Choice.

How Can Health Care Insurance Be Eliminated?

It may be unconstitutional or at least un-American to outlaw health care insurance. It would be more appropriate to legislate that health care insurance plans should be primary payers, and that Balanced Choice would be secondary, only paying after health care plans paid their full amount. This would make health care insurance financially unreasonable. In essence, health care insurance would no longer lower the consumer's portion of health care expense, but it would only lower the portion paid by Balanced Choice.

Employee retraining and an insurance buyout might be necessary

Eliminating health care insurance would benefit many people but it would cause unemployment for many workers in the health care insurance industry. Some of the insurance employees could be retrained to provide jobs delivering health care to the millions who were previously uninsured or to providing prevention and educational services. The lowered health care expenses would be an economic stimulus for American businesses, and this would provide additional jobs. Establishment of a safety net for unemployed insurance industry workers would be appropriate.

It is difficult to decide what to do with the stockholders of insurance companies. They might redirect their resources with a creative business plan that allows them to thrive in another area. In a capitalist society, some industries become obsolete and this is part of the risk investors take. Typewriter companies and horse buggy companies have faded or retooled when technology has made them obsolete.

On the other hand, the insurance industry has great power and influence, and it may be necessary for the government to give it financial compensation. A buyout would be less expensive then the continued government subsidies and wasted consumer dollars that are used to support this obsolete industry. A buy out, however, is a political question, and ultimately, the American people need to decide if and how much they will pay to remove the elephant from health care reform.

Conclusion

The insurance industry is huge. It could be considered the owner of health care. However, it does not effectively accomplish the goal of health care security and does not add enough value to justify its financial burden on the American people and employers. It is obsolete, and in any real health care reform proposal, it needs to go. Programs can be developed to address the needs of the employees and owners of the insurance industry.

Chapter 11–Patching Up
Insurance-Driven Health Care

Summary: Health care insurance advocates have numerous proposals for patching-up the system by expanding insurance coverage, usually with government subsidies. To conserve money, these proposals almost always include a provision for increasing the management of health care. There is a sharp difference of opinion on the desirability of more managed care; generally speaking, those who manage think it is a good solution, and those who are managed—providers and consumers— have a negative opinion. Other proposals call for conserving money by increasing cost-sharing in a manner that has some similarities to Balanced Choice. A number of proposals have been offered to address the needs of the uninsured. These include Medical Savings Accounts or consumer-driven models, mandatory insurance purchase, and universal health care vouchers. Many of these proposals have some of the ideas contained in Balanced Choice, but are not nearly as effective as Balanced Choice in solving problems in the health care system. None of the patch up proposals overcome the inherent dysfunctions in an insurance-driven health care system. All of the proposals to expand health insurance increase the NHE, instead of decreasing it as Balanced Choice does.

As the health care crisis escalates, numerous proposals are emerging to repair the damaged insurance-driven health care system. Some proposals address the increasing costs of health care by either looking for ways to increase managed care or asking consumers to increase cost sharing. Other proposals are designed to address the needs of the uninsured by expanding insurance coverage, which also increases the NHE. Although none of these ideas overcome the underlying problems in the insurance-driven health care system, it is worthwhile to examine the pros and cons of each idea.

Controlling Costs by Increasing Managed Care

Many economists think that with time, patients and providers will get used to third-party managers limiting their health care choices. They believe that increased managed care is inevitable; that it is the only way to control costs. Because they are on the side of managing the care are not being managed, they believe that managed care is desirable.

There is no doubt that managed care can provide adequate health care. Kaiser Permanente is probably the best example of how health care can be delivered through managed care. Many people who can only afford Kaiser are pleased to have some health care, and certainly prefer Kaiser to their status as uninsured. However, when most people have a choice, they want health care coverage that is less restrictive. As a nation that is spending 47% more per capita for health care than any other country, the people should get something better than Kaiser if it is possible.

There are many reasons why managed care has not created the efficient and high-quality systems that it has promised. Chapter 2, "A Health Care Economics Roadmap: Understanding Health Care Economics," describes the economic problems with managed care. Its large administrative expenses divert financial resources from the actual delivery of health care. Managed care does not sell its products in a marketplace where consumers have a real choice to change companies. Moreover, choice of which HMO or managed care entity to use is quite different than the kind of choices offered by Balanced Choice where patients can choose any provider, choose to switch one provider without having to change insurance company, and choose any appropriate treatment option, not just the ones offered by the HMO or managed care company.

A serious problem with managed care is the providers' conflicts of interest between patients and insurance companies. All managed care requires that providers have some degree of covert obligation to a managed care entity, which may result in *invisible rationing*—limiting patients to less expensive treatment options without informing them that additional or alternative treatment might be beneficial.[49]

Managed care advocates propose that by implementing advanced management techniques, managed care will lower costs, become efficient, offer high quality services, and no longer operate as a barrier to necessary health care. They offer three types of solutions for making managed care better—more aggressively managing care to lower costs, imposing evidence-based treatment guidelines, and developing measures that hold managed care accountable for better quality and outcome results.

More aggressively managing care

In theory, managed care is designed to direct patients into the most efficient and effective treatment. Many proposals suggest that patients can be enrolled in HMOs that will control costs by going beyond the routine selection of the best treatment and aggressively managing care to reduce costs. Under aggressive managed care, the choice of treatment option is strongly influenced by cost. The term "aggressive managed care" is actually a euphemism for invisible rationing. Such proposals can result in substandard health care services and are not a desirable solution.

Development of evidence-based medicine guidelines

Some propose that managed care companies could improve health care by implementing state-of-the-art evidence-based medicine guidelines. These guidelines would eliminate waste by focusing providers on proven and effective treatments.

The development of evidence-based medicine, as described in Chapter 8, "Science, Education, and Consumer Advocacy," is a good idea. When the science is clear and persuasive, evidence-based treatment guidelines can create a standard of practice for all providers. When the science is clear, providers will need to provide treatment according to current standards or risk malpractice. Management is not needed to enforce these non-controversial guidelines.

Since the beginning of managed care, companies have developed guidelines for care, and claimed that these guidelines were based on science. There is nothing new about managed care's role in guidelines now that they are called "evidence-based." The only way that managed care can use guidelines to reduce costs is to implement guidelines that go beyond the non-controversial accepted guidelines and into controversial areas. These guidelines are developed in proprietary secrecy and are not open to discussion from opposing points of view. The managed care employees who prepare guidelines not only look at science, but they also put an undisclosed emphasis on reducing costs so that the value of the science may be outweighed by concern about cost. Guidelines can result in bureaucratic medicine that is not responsive to individual differences, complex conditions, and/or a patient's personal preferences.

Balanced Choice recognizes the potential contribution of science and evidence-based medicine to improved health care. Balanced Choice proposes ways to introduce these advances without the rigid guidelines of managed care. Balanced Choice programs contribute to the distribution of evidence-based medical information to improve treatment options and to inform providers and consumers—not to restrict coverage.

Measures and data that will increase accountability for quality and outcomes

For several decades, managed care proponents have claimed that market competition will cause managed care companies to compete based on quality. The Clinton proposal for national health care was based on this idea and was called "Managed Competition." Theoretically, if managed care companies gave consumers improved quality or greater value, the companies would be rewarded with a larger market share. In this vision, competition results in managed care becoming an excellent, high-quality and efficient system of health care delivery with many satisfied customers.

This blissful vision has not come to pass. Analysts have correctly pointed out that one reason for the failure of managed care to live up to its promise is that there has not been a way to compare quality between companies. These analysts propose new ways to gather data on quality, outcome, and patient health. Accordingly, they argue that if the quality data is available, informed purchasers would be able to compare managed care companies and make choices based on quality. High quality companies would prosper and those that did not maintain quality would not survive.

Many of these ideas for data analysis are undoubtedly beneficial. All of health care can benefit from better outcome studies, improved quality measures, and an emphasis on health rather than illness. These new forms of data can lead to better health care. Designing and implementing quality and outcome-measurement systems, however, is easier said than done. So far, these measurement systems are not able to guide large health care bureaucracies towards high-quality care. Even with improved quality and outcome data, managed care would continue to be a rigid and cumbersome bureaucratic system that restricts health care choices.

Controlling Costs by Increasing Cost Sharing

When managed care was created, it promoted its ability to keep patient fees low. Its proponents argued that consumers should be charged a token copay because if charges were substantial, consumers might forego necessary as well as unnecessary care. Managed care proponents claimed that consumers were incapable of responsible cost-consciousness in health care issues. They argued that consumers, worried about their health, would blindly pay any price without considering cost, which would continue to contribute to cost escalation in health care. They argued that the only hope for controlling costs was an independent entity, managed care, that would prudently compare the value of services and strive for lower costs. Ironically, as managed care evolves, there is an increasing emphasis on asking consumers to assure a larger share of the cost of care so that they become cost conscious.

Pharmacy tiers are commonly used to make consumers sensitive to the difference in medication costs. Copayments are rising. In particular, expensive imaging tests may have substantial copayments to motivate consumers to ask their providers if the test is absolutely necessary. Deductibles are larger. To motivate patients to stay in-network, they are required to pay higher copayments if they choose an out-of-network provider.

Insurance and managed care companies are making some moves in the direction of Balanced Choice. They are using cost sharing (meaning patients pay a larger portion of the charges) to make consumers cost conscious. Balanced Choice, however, remains more effective in using cost consciousness to control health care expenses. Balanced Choice is not just sensitive to gross price differences between tiers, but it is also sensitive to small price differences and small price increases. Balanced Choice also makes cost information more available to patients at the place where they are making their treatment choices, in the provider's office. The question is, if cost consciousness is restored to consumers, what is the need for managed care?

Proposals for Reducing the Number of Uninsured with Expanded Insurance-Driven Health Care

Medical Savings Accounts (MSAs) and consumer-driven health care

MSAs, which are also called consumer-driven health care, have been proposed both as ways to reduce the number of uninsured and as a way to restructure the financing of health care. Consumer-driven health care is a label that describes systems in which consumers are given an income tax deduction for putting part of their income in a savings account that is reserved for medical expenses. In addition, consumers purchase insurance policies that cover catastrophic expenses but have high deductibles (several thousand dollars). Because consumers are spending their own money from the savings account for the first several thousand dollars, it is argued that they will be cost conscious about expenses, and therefore, there is no need for managed care. In addition, because the costs of administering the savings accounts and the high-deductible policy are less than a traditional insurance plan, there is some reduction in the administrative costs of insurance. Consumer-driven health care is touted as a way to provide health care security while returning market power to consumers and eliminating managed care.

Consumer-driven health care offers individuals with substantial incomes another way to reduce taxes and allows insurance companies or the banking system to gain profits from operating the health care savings accounts. Consumer driven health care advocates argue that it is only fair that consumers should be able to set up their own health plan with pre-tax dollars because employers are allowed to provide health care insurance as a pre-tax benefit. Unfortunately, there are several reasons that consumer-driven health care does little to help fix the health care system.

First, it is usually the high-income individuals who have extra income for a savings account for future medical problems. The tax break is most beneficial to the wealthy because they are in the highest tax bracket. In general though, high-income people already receive good health care. Giving them a tax break does little to fix the health care system, and at the same time, it reduces tax revenue that is needed to pay for tax-financed health care.

Second, today's health care system makes cost comparison very difficult. In fact, because it is so difficult to obtain comparable price information from providers, individuals often end up paying the highest cost for services. Providers, who have been pressured into discounting their services for large insurance companies, frequently recover their loses by charging self-pay patients the highest fees. It is not unusual for the self-pay patient to pay up to 64% more than someone who has a negotiated discount.[50]

Third, chronically ill patients and people with serious health conditions cannot purchase individual consumer-driven health care polices. Individuals still need to go through the expensive underwriting process, which results in excluding those with serious and chronic illnesses. Even if these individuals were not excluded by underwriters, the ongoing care for their chronic illnesses usually keeps these individuals from having spare income to put in a savings account. Their illnesses would continuously consume their savings accounts.

Fourth, consumer-driven health care still uses the obsolete insurance system for catastrophic expenses. This causes price escalation and undermines consumer cost consciousness for serious illnesses.

The beneficial aspect of MSAs and consumer-driven health care is that it restores consumer cost consciousness, just as Balanced Choice does. Unfortunately, consumer-driven health care remains a system that is primarily good for the healthy and wealthy, does not establish ways for consumers to compare costs, and it does not fix the underlying problems in the insurance-driven health care system.

Required insurance purchase

Some proposals suggest that the country could move closer to universal coverage by requiring everyone to purchase health insurance, just as people are required to purchase automobile insurance. To make this purchase affordable, these proposals usually suggest a federal subsidy to help pay for insurance plans.

Some of these proposals offer a basic health care plan that everyone can join for the same price regardless of age or health condition. Others suggest that the subsidies be "risk-adjusted" so that although people with health conditions or older people would pay more, they would also receive a larger subsidy.

It is difficult to imagine how to enforce compliance in such a system. In spite of laws requiring insurance for automobile registration and severe penalties, including jail time, for noncompliance, there are still a large number of uninsured motorists. Low-income people who cannot afford insurance are frequently the ones who do not purchase automobile insurance. Health care insurance costs more than automobile insurance, which suggests noncompliance would be an even greater problem. It is difficult to imagine how the very poor, those who cannot even afford a car, would be able to purchase the required health care insurance. In addition to uninsured motorists, there would continue to be problems with the medically uninsured. Would the medically uninsured be refused treatment at emergency rooms in these proposals? Who would pay their bills? Would they be fined or jailed as uninsured motorists can be? Would there be yet another health care payment system for the uninsured?

Universal health care vouchers

Some proposals suggest a federally funded universal health care voucher for basic care. Individuals could select from competing basic managed health care plans, and those who fail to select a plan could have one assigned to them. People who could afford more than the basic plan could choose to apply their subsidy to a higher quality plan.

These proposals would create a potential for the worst of the two-tiered systems. Because the amount of the voucher would put a cap on funds available, the basic managed care plans would be forced into managing care as aggressively as necessary to stay within the budget cap. The result could easily be extensive visible and invisible rationing for those who relied on the basic managed care packages.

These proposals give consumers some choice, but the choice is of limited value. People would have a voucher that allows them to choose which basic managed care plan to join. However, Dr. Jed Shapiro who provides services to people in jail says, "Inmates agree that some jails are better than others, but given a real choice, they would rather not be in any of them." One aggressively managed HMO can seem slightly better than another with the same budget cap per patient; however, are HMOs the best the

United States can provide when it spends 47% more per capita than the next highest spender?

The choice of a health care plan is difficult even for those who are fortunate enough to be able to purchase a more expensive plan. Plans are enormous and complex bundles of services. Most people have difficulty accurately understanding the true coverage and limitations. Even if current coverage is understood, plans can change their network of providers and internal regulations at any point. Once patients have chosen their plans, they could be stuck with the unforeseen consequences. If they have pre-existing conditions, changing plans can be difficult or prohibitively expensive. Real choice is choice of provider and each treatment option, not a choice of which insurance plan a person might get locked into.

Universal voucher proposals incorporate two of the benefits of Balanced Choice. First, they provide universal coverage. Second, they recognize that people should be able to pay for increased services, should they so choose, and providers should be able to determine their own fees.

Compared to Balanced Choice, both voucher and mandated purchase of basic insurance proposals lack several important features. They do not have a mechanism like the Mandatory Funding Split to maintain quality in the basic managed health care plans. They do not allow the full choice either of provider or treatment offered by Balanced Choice. And, they are much more expensive because they continue to subsidize the obsolete insurance industry with its expensive overhead costs.

Lowering the cost of insurance by eliminating government mandates and protections

As the costs of health care insurance rise, some are proposing that the number of uninsured could be reduced if government mandates for full coverage were eliminated. Other proposals call for allowing small employers from different states to group together and offer plans that would not need to meet the requirements of state laws. These are really proposals for offering partial-coverage health care insurance.

Theoretically, employers who have not insured their employees would decide to insure employees in one of these partial coverage plans. In reality though, employers are not acting eager to expand the number of employees that they are insuring, but quite the opposite. Employers are tending to decrease the number of people that they insure and wanting to decrease health care insurance expenses. Although a few employers who previously did not insure employees might purchase these partial-coverage plans, there might be many more who previously provided full coverage who might switch to the partial-coverage plans.

These are proposals that seem to lack any redeeming qualities. A person with partial coverage is underinsured. These proposals offer a way that a small decrease in the number of uninsured could be traded for a larger increase in the number of underinsured. This does not sound like forward progress.

Conclusion

Some of the attempts to patch up insurance-driven health care contain or strive toward features that are included in Balanced Choice. Many patches strive to decrease the number of uninsured, and some patches might almost achieve universal coverage. Many insurance plans allow out-of-network coverage at a higher cost to the consumer, which is similar to the Independent Plan in Balanced Choice. Cost sharing is being used to restore consumer cost consciousness. Along with cost sharing, consumers are being offered more choice. It adds validity to the Balanced Choice proposal that insurance proposals incorporate some of Balanced Choice's features, even if insurance is incorporating these features on a limited basis.

There are three main drawbacks to these proposals. First, none of them overcome the numerous dysfunctions of insurance-driven health care described in Chapter 10, "Health Care Insurance is Obsolete." Second, as consumer cost consciousness is increasingly being used to hold down the cost of health care, and insurance-driven health care offers less real consumer choice than Balanced Choice, there is little value to maintaining the insurance-driven health care system. Third, the patch-up proposals that make progress toward fixing problems in the health care system each require a large increase in expenditures. If these proposals do not fix the basic problem, insurance does not add value, and the proposals will cost more money, what good are they?

116

In essence, these patch-up proposals are ways that the government and taxpayers are being asked to subsidize the health care insurance industry. The patches don't fix the underlying problems, insurance-driven health care doesn't add value, and it makes health care too expensive. Even with patches, insurance is the elephant in the health care reform room.

Chapter 12–Balanced Choice
Compared to Single Payer

Summary: Single payer proposals are superior to the efforts to patch up the insurance-driven health care systems, and both single payer systems and Balanced Choice solve many of the same problems. Balanced Choice, however, has more advantages than single payer proposals. Balanced Choice maintains consumer cost consciousness, and consequently does not require managing care. Single payer systems, on the other hand, undermine cost consciousness and require some management to prevent over-utilization of services. Single payer systems control costs by having the government control fees while Balanced Choice offers providers more choices about setting fees. Balanced Choice has more incentives for encouraging improved quality and innovation. It has greater potential for gaining support from consumers, providers, and employers. In many ways, Balanced Choice can be conceptualized as an enhanced single payer system that overcomes the drawbacks to a single payer system.

Both single payer proposals and Balanced Choice solve many problems in health care financing. Both establish universal coverage. Both provide free services to the very low-income patients and those with catastrophic health care expenses. Both relieve employers of the burden of high and escalating costs for health care, workers compensation, and motor vehicle insurance. Both create a system that can capture the benefits of prevention. Both have cost-containment mechanisms. Most importantly, both lower expenses by eliminating the costly administration of the insurance and managed care industries.

Single payer systems have a proven track record in countries around the world. Many countries with single payer systems rate better than the United States on measures of infant mortality, longevity and treatment outcomes.[51] There are many reasonable and good people who are promoting single payer systems because of moral, ethical, financial or medical reasons. Many single payer advocates may prefer Balanced Choice as they understand that it addresses most of their concerns and offers important advantages.

Amount of Choice

Consumers' choices

An advantage of single payer systems is that they appear to give consumers choice of provider or treatment without the burden of the gap payment. In single payer proposals, a small copay is usually all that is required for treatment. This freedom from concerns about cost unfortunately has a hidden consequence that, in effect, can decrease choice. If consumers do not need to worry about cost, they lose cost consciousness. As the insurance-driven health care system has shown, someone needs to manage costs. In addition to the government setting fees, single payer systems would need to institute extensive managed care to control costs, just as insurance-driven health care has needed managed care. Thus, a single payer system would become a large unitary managed care system, and it would restrict choice for consumers.

Providers' choices

In single payer systems, fees are set through government negotiations with provider groups. There is one fee schedule and providers are not allowed to charge more than the government fee. For this reason, many providers are vehemently opposed to a single payer system. Providers have had experience with Medicaid and Medicare setting reimbursement fees so low that, if they accept many Medicare or Medicaid patients, they cannot financially sustain their practices. Providers do not want to trust their futures to a system in which the government can set rigid reimbursement rates. Moreover, the independent providers in the United States do not want to join together in a union-like arrangement in order to negotiate rates or to have to consider striking if negotiations failed.

Balanced Choice: Choice for both

In single payer proposals, consumer choice of provider is given priority over the provider's choice of how much to charge for services. Balanced Choice is a compromise between consumers and providers; it balances consumer choices with provider choices rather than giving higher priority to one group's choices. Consumers have full range of choices if they are willing to pay the gap payment. Providers have the choice of accepting the government fee on the Standard Plan, setting their own fees on the Independent Plan, or participating in both plans.

Cost Containment Mechanisms

Single payer systems have the power to control costs by setting the fees for all services. This power to set fees, the power of a monopsony, is an effective cost-control mechanism. The danger, however, in a single payer system is that if reimbursements are set too low, there will eventually be a shortage of providers, quality will decrease, and less incentive for innovation will gradually erode medical advances.

Balanced Choice encourages quality and innovation. If the Standard Plan reimbursements are too low for providers to offer quality care, more providers and consumers will choose to move to the Independent Plan, where higher reimbursement would allow for improved quality. The Mandatory Funding Split would then require that Balanced Choice respond by increasing the amount of reimbursements for the Standard Plan. The higher reimbursements would attract providers back to the Standard Plan and restore quality. In other words, when quality starts to decline in Balanced Choice, there is an automatic mechanism that restores funding and quality to the part of the system that has set reimbursements.

The ability to profit from innovation is a powerful incentive for advances in medicine. Reducing cost is essential, but it is only part of creating the optimal health care system. Both single payer and Balanced Choice are effective in lowering the cost of established treatment. In the single payer system, costs are lowered because the government can negotiate a lower price. In Balanced Choice, the gap payments create consumer cost consciousness, which lowers price. In Balanced Choice, however, innovations that improve health care can be charged at a higher price—whatever the market will bear. The manufacturer does not need to fear that the government will set reimbursements so low that it undermines the incentive for innovation. For example, a pharmaceutical company with a medication that is either more effective or has fewer side effects can charge a higher price (thus creating a larger gap payment) and still attract consumers. Because manufacturers could gain financial rewards for innovation, they would maintain their incentive to develop better medications.

Potential Stakeholder and Political Support

Although there have been many surveys that show broad support for a single payer system, to this point, the support has not been sustained when it has been challenged. Sometimes voters agree with the concept but not the details of single payer proposals, and other times the opponents, including many providers and many employers, dissuade the American people from their support for a single payer proposal.

Even when proponents of single payer proposals cite the quality health care available in countries with single payer systems, the opponents argue that the United States could not have a quality government-run system. In health care, the three largest government-run programs are Medicare, Medicaid and the Veterans Administration. Each of these systems has had numerous problems. Even in Medicare, which has been the best of the three, there have been times that reimbursement rates have been so low that providers could not afford to take additional Medicare patients and remain in business. So many providers fear the restrictions and bureaucracy of a government-run, single payer system that such a system is unlikely to win the necessary political support.

The opinions of employers are also very important. Without the enthusiastic support of employers, there is little chance that there will be enough political pressure to overcome the power of the insurance lobby, which will oppose any movement away from insurance-driven health care. Employers are unlikely to endorse a single payer proposal because they usually are more aligned philosophically with conservative and market philosophies. They are more likely to support a Balanced Choice proposal because it provides the option of choosing from two Plans, and it uses market forces rather than government regulation to keep the system functioning effectively.

The question is not whether the government should be involved in health care. Indeed, 60% of the funds for health care currently come from the government.[52] Almost all proposals to fix health care involve an increase in government funding. Even the conservative and insurance-driven proposals ask for the government to subsidize individual insurance plans. There is general agreement that increased government funding is needed to fix the health care system. The question is whether the stakeholders will accept using increased government funding for a single payer system because it means having rules and fees set by the government-run system. Without the option of the Independent Plan, it is unlikely that direct government funding for universal health care would be adopted.

Although single payer plans are viable in many countries, the political situation in the United States makes a single payer system unlikely. To gain the support of providers and employers, as well as the largest possible consensus of consumers, a system that allows more choice and less government restriction is needed. Balanced Choice is such a system.

Maintaining Quality Throughout the System

Single payer advocates argue that they can assure that everyone has quality health care. They are concerned that any two-tiered system will result in somewhat inferior treatment on the lower tier, and that eventually such a system will result in substandard care for the poor and disabled. Indeed, inadequate care for low-income people is likely in the insurance-driven proposals for two-tiered or multi-tiered systems.

It is not altogether true that single payer systems have only one tier, and that everyone will obtain the same health care. While these systems attempt to legislate only one system, the wealthy always find a way to obtain better care than others. All single payer systems in the world have a way that the wealthy can obtain more services, special services, or if all else fails, they can leave the country for services in another country.

The Standard Plan in Balanced Choice would not become substandard care for the poor as single payer advocates fear. The Mandatory Funding Split maintains sufficiently high reimbursements for Standard Plan providers so that providers would choose to accept Standard Plan patients at least half of the time. Likewise, consumers would often choose to use the Standard Plan, even when they can afford the Independent plan because it would offer quality service. This freedom of movement from one Plan to the other, for providers and consumers, is so fluid that Balanced Choice accurately describes them as "Plans" rather than tiers.

The boundaries dividing the Standard and Independent Plans are not rigid, as they are in many other proposals. Most providers will have patients on both the Standard Plan and the Independent Plan, and most consumers will use the Standard Plan on some occasions and the Independent Plan on other occasions. The overlap of consumers and providers in the Standard Plan and Independent Plan will blur the distinction between the two "tiers."

Single payer proponents suggest that to maintain quality health care for all, the decision-makers should have the same health care coverage as the average person. Quite accurately, they note that in the current system decision-makers—politicians, business owners, insurance executives, and managers of health care—have excellent insurance plans while many people in the system are restricted by aggressive managed care, are uninsured, or are underinsured. As long as there are two distinct tiers or multiple tiers, decision makers and the politically powerful will be in the upper tier and will lose their sensitivity to the lower tiers.

Although Balanced Choice allows for different levels of care, the two Plans are always kept in balance with each other through the 60/40 Mandatory Funding Split. The split assures that decision-makers and the politically powerful cannot change the quality of one Plan without changing the quality of the other. There is only one system. The participants in Independent Plan cannot benefit from increased funding and services unless it is balanced by increases in funding and services for the Standard Plan. No one group benefits unless the other benefits. If more funds or resources are needed for health care, politically, both the users of the Standard Plan and the Independent Plan will need to work together.

For-Profit Versus Not-for-Profit Medicine

Many single payer proposals call for the end of "for-profit medicine." These demands are philosophically and economically confusing. Throughout health care, providers are working for their own profit, whether as owners of their practice or on salary. Manufacturers of medical supplies and medications are for-profit enterprises. Single payer advocates are not asking that providers and manufacturers stop working for profit, but are usually saying that the people who control health care decisions (e.g., managed care companies) should not make a profit from restricting health care. Instead of for-profit management of health care, single payer proposals require government management to set reimbursements and control overuse. Balanced Choice proponents agree; they do not believe that managed care entities should make a profit from limiting health care. In Balanced Choice there are no for-profit managed care entities.

Conclusion

Balanced Choice can be seen as an enhanced single payer system. Balanced Choice provides most of the same advantages of a single payer system and overcomes the disadvantages. By adding the Independent Plan, Balanced Choice has fewer restrictions. Gap payments maintain consumer cost consciousness, which eliminates the need for most managed care. Balanced Choice has more incentives to improve quality and encourage innovation. Most importantly, it has more potential to gain support from consumers, providers, and employers.

Chapter 13–Solid Advantages with Balanced Choice: A Reply to Skepticism

Summary: Balanced Choice challenges traditional assumptions about health care. Skeptics may doubt the ability of consumers to be responsibly involved in health care and question whether market forces can control the rising cost of health care. There are, however, practical and common sense reasons to believe that such an innovative system is feasible. In response to each skeptic's question, reasons are presented to show that Balanced Choice is a solid system that offers more promise than other proposals.

Balanced Choice challenges some of the common assumptions about health care systems. Many experts have assumed that consumers cannot take a responsible role in health care decisions. Balanced Choice places consumers in a central decision-making role. It is conventional wisdom that the health care market does not respond to market dynamics, and therefore, containing the escalating costs of health care requires management and regulation. Balanced Choice strives to restore market dynamics. It has also been accepted thinking that the only available choices are single payer or insurance-driven health care. Balanced Choice is a feasible third choice.

Predictably, there is skepticism whenever basic assumptions are challenged. Upon examination, however, even skeptics will find that there is good reason to believe that consumers can take an active role in health care decisions, that market forces can be used to contain costs, and that Balanced Choice is indeed an alternative that is advantageous.

Can Consumers Responsibly Take an Active Role in Health Care Decisions?

Can consumers make responsible decisions about cost?

Greater consumer involvement in cost decisions is being encouraged throughout health care. Insurance companies are moving toward increasing cost sharing and increasing the amount of copays. Pharmaceuticals are commonly on a tier system to encourage consumers to select less expensive medications, and patients do respond to this cost information when it is available.[53] MSAs and consumer-driven health care plans use consumer cost consciousness as the only cost-control mechanism. It is becoming generally accepted that consumers can and need to be more involved in cost decisions.

Balanced Choice not only gives patients the opportunity to make cost-conscious decisions, but more so than any other proposal, it establishes methods for giving consumers the necessary information for cost comparisons. It establishes cost-comparison information for pharmaceuticals, provides a method for comparing costs of lab and imaging tests, and creates a method for comparing the charges of various providers in the Independent Plan. Balanced Choice makes this information available to providers so that they also can consider cost in their recommendations.

Consumers do not need to be medical experts to make decisions about cost. Consumers gather information from experts, evaluate that information, and make their decisions. Providers would still prescribe, determine the treatment that is essential, and explain the treatment options. Because cost information is available to consumers when they make health care decisions, and because they can consult with a provider about the benefits of various choices, they can make wise decisions, as they do with other purchases.

Should patients and providers spend valuable treatment time talking about costs?

Somebody in the health care system needs to be concerned about the cost of treatment. If it is not the patients and providers, then it will need to be managed care or a government-managed health care system. Once managers are involved, patients and providers spend valuable treatment time talking about what the managed care system allows. In order for patients and providers to maintain control over treatment decisions, they need to incorporate time for a discussion of costs.

Patients ultimately have responsibility for their own health care, including their investment of time and money. Balanced Choice advocates it is better to emphasize this personal responsibility than to avoid it.

Isn't Balanced Choice too complicated for patients?

Balanced Choice is much less complicated than the current system. In the current system, patients need to make choices about which insurance plan they will need to purchase. Insurance plans have enormously complex bundles of benefits. It is difficult for anyone to decipher these packages. Much of the information about how the plan will be managed is proprietary, and if it were available, it might make understanding the plans even more difficult. Finding the right plan requires predicting all future health care needs, an impossible task.

In Balanced Choice, decisions are not bundled and patients do not need to predict their future needs. Patients do not need to understand the whole system; they only need to understand information pertinent to each decision. Decisions are made one at a time, which is much easier than making bundled decisions. Patients need only choose which Plan they will use to find a provider, and the provider will present choices, one at a time.

Can gap payments limit unnecessary and encourage necessary tests and treatment?

It is often a matter of opinion whether or not treatment or tests are necessary. Managed care presumes that bureaucratic utilization review and proprietary guidelines will result in the best decisions about what is necessary. Patients and providers would disagree, and they have many examples of how managed care can be too restrictive. Unless there is a consensus in the medical community that a specific treatment is unnecessary and wasteful, treatment decisions will not be clear-cut, and who the decision-makers are will become important. Balanced Choice believes that providers and patients are the right team for making health care decisions.

Many treatment decisions are not clear-cut; there is some personal discretion about how necessary the treatment is. The reason for requiring gap payments is to avoid having providers and/or patients say, "I do not care about cost or if the treatment is necessary because insurance is paying the bill." Gap payments encourage patients to ask, "How necessary is this treatment? Is there a less expensive way to find the information needed? How much do the recommended treatment options cost?" When providers are aware that cost is a concern to the patient, they can consider cost as a factor in their recommendations. With this awareness, the provider-patient team can be effective in limiting unnecessary interventions and in utilizing only necessary tests and treatment.

Is management needed to assure that monies are spent on quality health care that provides effective outcomes?

Many people believe that management oversight is the best way to assure that there is an emphasis on outcomes and quality. Theoretically, the central control offered by a managed care company can demand better outcomes, pay for results, and require higher quality. In practice, managed care companies are more concerned about cost than about improved quality of medical services. Improved quality is certainly not the experience of the vast majority of patients and providers.

What is needed is better information, not more management. As more information is available about quality and outcomes, informed consumers will ask providers for this information. Information about health care is continuously available, now including information from the Internet, and informed consumers increasingly ask their providers important questions about quality and outcome. Consumers, as the recipients of health care, are invested in quality and outcome as well as cost. Managed care, which is not a recipient health care, is overly concerned about financial matters. There is no reason to doubt that informed consumers would be able to improve quality and outcome as well or better than managed care.

Can Balanced Choice Control the Rising Cost of Health Care?

Does Balanced Choice address the increasing cost of health care that stems from medical advances and an aging population?

Medical advances and an aging population are increasing the cost of health care, both in actual dollars and in percentage of Gross Domestic Product (GDP). This creates unsolved problems for all health care proposals. The only proposals that address this issue are the ones that call for aggressively managing care to the point of rationing or for discouraging medical advances.

It is a mistake to think that a health care system should first look for ways to ration care or slow advances of medicine. The first question should be, "Is the system delivering health care to Americans in the most efficient manner?" It is clear that under the current mess of 17 different systems,

America is not getting the most health care possible for the amount being spent. Adopting Balanced Choice will not only make the system work so that everyone can have health care security, but it makes the system more efficient.

Balanced Choice makes established health care treatments less expensive so that there is more money available for medical advances. The ways Balanced Choice could lower the cost of established medications (which are actually rising in the current system) were explained in Chapter 7, "A Balanced Choice Pharmacy Plan." With the savings in treatment, medications, and administration, money is available to fund research that furthers the development of less expensive treatments.

Even with lowering the costs of existing health care, many of the medical advances increase the cost of care, and that, combined with the increasing medical needs of an aging population, will require a larger share of the GDP. There is, however, nothing sacred about the percentage of GDP that is spent on health care. In other areas of consumer expense, it is the market that determines what percentage of GDP is spent on food, transportation, housing, electronics, or recreation. It is assumed that only consumers can decide whether it is better to spend money on one area rather than another. In general, many people think that if better health were possible for more years of their lives, then it would be worth spending more of the GDP. In its final proposal, Balanced Choice, like any system, will need a plan for increasing revenue to cover the predictable cost increases.

Does the Independent Plan work with hospital and specialty-care costs?

Hospital costs, surgeries, and some specialty care are expensive. Can consumers really afford to pay a percentage of these costs on the Independent Plan? The market is already answering the question. Insurance is creating plans that have different hospital tiers, each requiring patients to pay a different percentage of the hospital bill as coinsurance.[54] Consumers who purchase a catastrophic health care plan often expect to pay the first $5,000 or more of health care expenses. People pay $5,500 for braces for their children. Because most people usually have a limited number of operations and hospitalizations, it is not unreasonable to expect that many would choose to pay several thousand dollars for the ability to use the Independent Plan for a hospitalization or operation.

Although some patients could afford and would choose the Independent Plan for hospitalization and provider, it is probable that some expensive procedures, some specialties, and extended hospital stays might have a smaller portion of patients choosing the Independent Plan than Standard Plan.

What can Balanced Choice do about high-cost procedures?

A vexing problem for the future of health care is the impact of high-cost procedures. Medical advances offer more and more expensive ways to treat illness and prolong life. Balanced Choice offers a more efficient system that can cover all necessary health care now and in the short-term future. There is likely to be a point, however, when the high-cost options will be too much for Balanced Choice or any other system to cover.

Imagine, for example, the invention of an artificial heart that costs $500,000. No health care system, including Balanced Choice, could afford to give this heart to every person who could use one. As the number of high-cost procedures increase, any health care system will need to consider rationing. Because Balanced Choice is an efficient system, it will postpone the question of rationing longer than other systems. At some point, however, rationing will need to be considered for new, high-cost procedures and at that time the decisions will be made openly, with public knowledge and input.

Is Balanced Choice a Feasible System?

Can a reasonable Standard Plan reimbursement schedule be established?

The initial Standard Plan reimbursement schedule easily can be based on the current Medicare reimbursement schedule. Only a few adjustments would be needed to make the Standard Plan reimbursement schedule acceptable to providers at least half of the time.

Is it too complicated to make the adjustments for the Mandatory Funding Split?

Providers and consumers do not need to understand how to make the Mandatory Funding Split adjustments in order to provide or receive health care. Only health care economists need to understand how to make the Mandatory Funding Split adjustments, and it is not that difficult. Health care economists could examine the data about the utilization of both Plans to determine if provider and consumer choices were resulting in the Mandated Funding Split. If the system were out of balance, the Balanced Choice Governing Board would make adjustments in either the Standard Plan reimbursement schedule or the Independent Plan reimbursement percentage. These adjustments have some similarity to adjustments that the Federal Reserve makes. After an adjustment, the data would be observed again to see if provider and consumer choices were resulting in the mandated split. If not, another adjustment would be made.

The reimbursement adjustments called for by the Mandatory Funding Split will have an effect on health care inflation, provider income, and available funds for medical advances. It will be important that Balanced Choice has methods, guidelines, and requirements for assuring that the average health care provider income will rise at the rate of inflation, that established treatments will decline in cost, and that funds are available to encourage improved and innovative treatment. While expensive medical advances and improved treatments may cause health care costs to rise more than the rate of general inflation, in Balanced Choice, these should be the only reasons that health care inflation exceeds general inflation.

Does Balanced Choice have the same disadvantages as school vouchers?

School vouchers are criticized because they can have a harmful effect on public schools. Voucher systems give each student the same amount of funds regardless of their individual educational needs. Students who are highly motivated and do not require extra resources (low-need students) might take their vouchers and disproportionately leave public school. This could lead to the public school having inadequate resources for the high-need students who remain.

In Balanced Choice, having patients leave the Standard Plan does not have the same effect on the system as school vouchers for several reasons. First, if the healthy (low-need) patients leave the Standard Plan, they only take with them enough funding to pay for their limited needs. Second, because the Independent Plan reimbursement percentage is less than 100%, Balanced Choice actually pays less for the people who use the Independent Plan. Thus, when patients use Balanced Choice payments for the Independent Plan, they do not deplete the resources for Standard Plan patients. Third, because the Mandatory Funding Split requires adjusting reimbursement schedules to maintain the 60/40 split, the Standard Plan always receives enough funds for the patients who choose the Standard Plan.

Is Balanced Choice a government-run system?

Balanced Choice is not a government-run health care system. It is merely a way to finance the private and independent providers who operate the health care system. Providers are not government employees and only receive part of their income from the Balanced Choice health care fund, with the remainder coming from patients. Unlike a traditional single payer system, providers can charge more than the Balanced Choice Standard Plan fees by using the Independent Plan.

Will Americans accept another tax?

Many Americans are categorically opposed to taxes. However, market advocates, single payer advocates, conservatives, and liberals all propose using tax money to finance health care. It is widely accepted that some form of taxation is necessary to fix the health care systems.

The choice is between paying higher costs for health care insurance in an insurance-driven health care system or paying less, on the average, for a Balanced Choice system funded through taxation. Do Americans want lower taxes offset by higher insurance premiums in a system where they could lose their health care coverage any time their employment situation changes? It is likely that total cost and how well the system works is more important to most people than whether they pay their money to an insurance company or make contributions to a Balanced Choice health care fund.

A Balanced Choice tax is not a tax that is used to support special interests or a segment of the population. It is a tax that will directly benefit all people and their family members each time that they need health care. The Social Security System is a similar government benefit, and it is generally supported. Likewise, Americans may accept a tax if it could provide an efficient health care security system for all. The voters should be given the choice.

Conclusion

Skeptics may question the ability of consumers to be responsibly involved in health care decisions, the ability of market forces to slow the rising cost of health care, and the feasibility of an innovative system. However, increased consumer involvement in health care decisions is the direction that health care systems are moving. As insurance and managed care have not been able to slow the rising cost of health care adequately, they are also moving toward using market forces. When compared to the alternative proposals, Balanced Choice is not only feasible, but it is also administratively simpler to implement.

Chapter 14–Traveling the Road to the Cure: Consumers, Providers, and Employers Lead

Summary: Balanced Choice is a package of interconnected features that if implemented as a whole is a reform proposal that can create an efficient and effective system for financing health care in the U.S. The power to reform health care comes from the combined strength of the stakeholder groups—consumers, providers, and employers. Balanced Choice has a five-phase plan for unifying consumers, providers, and employers in reforming the health care system. The first phase is describing the idea—the content of this book. Second is researching areas where information is incomplete, conducting a more specific analysis of Balanced Choice costs, and building an organization that can develop Balanced Choice. Third is developing alliances with stakeholders and adapting and modifying Balanced Choice to address the needs of stakeholders. Fourth is developing and promoting necessary legislation. And fifth is implementation.

Balanced Choice is a new way to finance our health care systems. It sets a new direction by combining the virtues of competing proposals into one system. This book describes how it can be done. With Balanced Choice it is possible to have one system that not only fits with the American values of freedom of choice for providers and patients, but also provides health care security for all.

Instead of looking for a short-term, patch-up fix, Balanced Choice proposes stepping back and looking for the development of an idea that will really work. The disadvantage of this approach is that it takes time to develop the ideas, to disseminate the ideas, and to inform enough people about the ideas so that they can be part of the discussion. The advantage, however, is that this approach might really work, and in the long run, thoughtful development through the five phases may be the fastest way to cure the health care system.

Essential Balanced Choice Features

Standard Plan

- Small copay or gap payment
- First two visits/year free
- Financial assistance
- Emergency care

Independent Plan

- Greater choice of providers
- Provider able to set fees
- Gap and base payment

Balanced By

- Affordable prices
- Price comparison
- Unbundled choice
- Mandatory Funding Split
- Choice of Plan for both patients and providers
- Independent Plan is reimbursed at less than 100% of the Standard Plan

Quality Maintained By

- Consumer Health Advocacy Organization
- Education is preferred method of regulation
- Medical advisors help patients make choices
- Balanced Choice is a financing system, not a regulatory system

Additional Benefits

- Universal coverage
- Reduced costs for employers
- Eliminates employer responsibility for health care
- Protects employers from future tax increases
- Rapid reimbursement

(This diagram and its features are explained in Appendix A.)

Balanced Choice needs to be implemented as a package.

Balanced Choice is a set of interconnected features that need to be established as a complete package in order to create an efficient and effective system for financing health care for the entire country. The features are synergistic in that together they are more effective than the sum of the benefits of each feature. While additional features may enhance Balanced Choice, the package presented here is essential to the Balanced Choice proposal. The Essential Balanced Choice Features diagram graphically displays how the features are interconnected and related.

The power required for reform

Balanced Choice does not avoid the elephant in the health care reform movement. Many of the problems in the health care systems of the United States stem from being based on insurance. Balanced Choice creates a system that makes insurance obsolete. While this is the best for the country, it will almost eliminate the health insurance industry, which will use all of its power and resources to oppose Balanced Choice.

Balanced Choice is not the only proposal that calls for eliminating the health care insurance industry. A Canadian-style single payer system would also replace health care insurance. Because single payer proposals have many supporters already, it is clear that many people are ready to eliminate the health insurance industry.

Balanced Choice has the potential to become a reality because it is beneficial to three important stakeholders—consumers, providers, and employers. Combined, these groups have the power to create health care reform and overcome the opposition of the health care insurance industry. Most importantly, because employers will gain so much financially, they can be motivated to donate resources and disseminate information to counter the well-financed opposition of the health insurance industry.

Is changing a health care system too big a task for the United States?
* Balanced Choice is not a proposal for changing the health care system; *Balanced Choice merely changes the financing of health care.* It eliminates the middleman system of health insurance. Providers are the heart, soul, and core of the system, and they would continue to deliver health care. Eliminating the health care

insurance industry is not that disruptive because it adds little value and causes many of the problems in health care delivery.

- In Medicare, the United States already has a program for financing health care. *The United States is not starting from scratch in developing a system for financing health care.* Although Medicare needs improvement, it offers a starting place for developing Balanced Choice.

The Five-Phase Plan for Reforming the U.S. Health Care Systems with Balanced Choice

Phase One—Describing a solution

This book is part of the first step in the plan. Before a new idea can be considered, it must be described with enough clarity so people understand how the new idea works—even when the new idea makes common sense. Usually people need to think about a new idea before they warm up to it. Usually there are questions and doubts that need to be addressed. People routinely approach an idea by looking for its weaknesses and probe for reasons it might not work. Skepticism is a normal and healthy response.

I hope this book has explained Balanced Choice well enough that readers can understand the basic ideas and enough questions have been answered that its potential is clear. The book does not need to be a conclusive argument that Balanced Choice, as currently envisioned, should be adopted immediately. Rather, it is intended to inspire the reader to believe that Balanced Choice is headed in the right direction. If the book is successful, a reader will understand Balanced Choice well enough to discuss it as a viable proposal for health care reform.

Phase Two—Building an organization and conducting research

The second phase involves long-range planning and building a foundation for Balanced Choice development. To demonstrate feasibility and accurately estimate costs, additional analysis is needed to detail the costs and savings involved in converting to Balanced Choice. It is also important in this phase to enlist advocates and collaborators who can help introduce Balanced Choice into the national discourse on health care reform.

More analysis, cost projections, and evaluations are needed to answer the following questions:

1. How much can be saved by the elimination of multiple insurance and managed care plans and by converting to Balanced Choice? This evaluation needs to include the direct savings from eliminating insurance plans as well as the indirect savings from eliminating the expenses that providers incur in working with these plans, the expenses that employers incur in managing health care plans, and the cost in time and money that consumers incur in dealing with these plans.

2. What is the projected cost of Balanced Choice for the next ten years and twenty-five years?

3. What level of funding will be required to maintain Balanced Choice for the next ten years and twenty-five years?

4. How much does consumer cost consciousness affect prices in health care? This question can be answered by examining areas of health care that are self-paid such as over the counter medications, eyeglasses, and orthodontics.

5. How well do gap payments lower costs? This question can be answered by looking at gap payments in the Australian health care system and at some European countries that use gap payments for medications.

6. How would out-of-pocket costs in Balanced Choice compare to current out-of-pocket expenses for consumers?

7. How would Balanced Choice affect different medical specialties? It is important to meet with representatives of provider groups to identify potential difficulties and possible solutions in Balanced Choice.

8. Would the Independent Plan be feasible for major surgery or extended hospitalization? If not, how would these be handled in Balanced Choice?

9. What are the costs of transitioning to Balanced Choice? This evaluation should take into consideration the possible retraining of employees in the obsolete insurance industry as well as the many employees of providers whose positions are devoted to working with managed care and insurance entities.

10. How much would transition to Balanced Choice affect employers? This evaluation includes the savings realized from eliminating employer responsibility for health care and the health-related costs of workers compensation. The evaluation would also include the impact on employers who currently do not contribute to health care.

Support during this phase comes from those who are willing and able to take a long-term perspective on health care reform. Not every potential supporter is in this position. Generally, politicians cannot support an idea that does not have an active support group or is not ready for legislation. The same is true for health care provider organizations and consumer-advocacy organizations. These organizations need to keep their attention focused on more immediate legislative possibilities. Politicians and these organizations also need to be careful about offending the insurance industry before there is substantial support from their constituents.

Supporters in the long-term planning phase may come from people in think tanks, columnists, retired politicians, leaders in the provider-advocate and consumer-advocate community, employers, and concerned individuals. These are the people who can aid by helping to bring Balanced Choice into the national health care discourse. The goals in this phase are to garner some support, provide a thorough analysis of the specific details of Balanced Choice, and familiarize the health care reform community with the ideas in Balanced Choice.

Phase Three—Alliance building and modifications

Although Balanced Choice is built on the advice and wisdom of many people, it is primarily the work of the author. One person can sometimes develop a more creative vision than a group can develop, and I believe that is the case with Balanced Choice. However, a proposal to change the health care system cannot be the product of one person's vision. To be successful, it needs to become the product of many people working together to provide the wisdom and knowledge needed to make it work. A working board and organization will be necessary to move Balanced Choice forward. Alliances can improve it. As more people become involved, it will be modified, and I will lose the single authorship status. As an evolving proposal, the authorship will move to a cooperative group. Even further down the road, if Balanced Choice should become the basis for health care in this country, ownership would transfer to the American people.

In this phase, it is important for Balanced Choice to build alliances with provider organizations and consumer advocate organizations. As these organizations join, they will undoubtedly have specific concerns and issues that require refinements or modifications of Balanced Choice. If Balanced Choice is to satisfy the interests of the stakeholder groups, it is essential to bring them into the planning process. These alliances will later be able to serve as the foundation for educating the public and for successful legislative action.

Phase Four—Mobilizing to make Balanced Choice a political reality

Before turning Balanced Choice over to the legislative process, it is important that it is developed to the point that does not need to be changed in order to obtain widespread support. The legislature is not the best place for developing innovative ideas, designing new programs, or creating a new health care system. Legislators change every two years and consequently tend toward short-term planning. When legislation is developed, it often looks like a Christmas tree with ornaments attached for every powerful lobbing group. This kind of piecemeal process is not a good way to create a new health care financing system. If, however, Balanced Choice can design a comprehensive proposal that has broad-based support, the legislative process will only need to make adjustments and refine the proposal.

The strength of Balanced Choice is that it has a design that is indeed in the best financial interests of consumers, providers, and employers, and that it combines the security of universal coverage with the use of market forces. In other words, it achieves the goals of liberals and conservatives. It is also the right thing to do because it provides good care for all people.

It is necessary to combine the power of these three groups to overcome the lucrative and powerful lobbies that will oppose Balanced Choice. The insurance industry is the primary opposition, and there may be opposition from other groups. To succeed, Balanced Choice needs the financial and political support of the business community.

Reforming the health care systems in the United States will require a different kind of political mobilization than typical legislative proposals. Reform cannot be just a Republican or Democrat issue. To be successful, it will require strong general support from voters and strong bipartisan support. An enormous amount of money may be needed to counter the resistance of the health insurance industry. It will need to be led by the stakeholders who are experiencing the health care crisis—consumers, providers, and employers.

The road to legislative success will be difficult. If, however, Balanced Choice does unite consumers, providers and employers, it can move forward. With adequate financial resources and the support of employers, provider groups, and consumer-advocacy groups, it would be possible to pass legislation that converted the multiple United States health care systems to Balanced Choice.

Phase Five—Implementing Balanced Choice

As Balanced Choice becomes a reality, transition will entail a few adjustments. Payment systems would need to be established, the previously uninsured would seek out treatment, and many of the employees of insurance companies would become unemployed.

Establishing payment systems should pose few difficulties. It would be possible to set up a payment system that had practice (dry runs) before the transition.

Providing treatment for the millions of previously uninsured could pose a substantial problem. Many of the uninsured forego treatment or postpone seeing a provider. If all of the uninsured became eligible for treatment on the same day, it could overwhelm the health care system. It may be necessary to prepare for several months of extraordinary high demand and system overload. The existence of this problem is a sad commentary on the plight of the uninsured.

When health care dollars are transitioned from the insurance industry to the delivery of health care, there will also be a transition of employment opportunity. Many employees of the obsolete insurance industry will become unemployed, and there will be new opportunities in health care. Adequate unemployment insurance and job retraining funds need to be made available. In addition, there would need to be a plan for training people for the new opportunities in health care once there is universal coverage.

Conclusion

Is it tilting at windmills to think that the health care systems in the United States could be cured? Some critics would say that it is too big a problem, too complicated, and too risky. They would say that solving the problems would create too many enemies. Such skepticism overlooks the many reasons that it is quite possible to cure the health care systems. The United States already spends more money than any other country without getting the same results as other countries. In spite of the huge expenses, one out of seven people do not have health care insurance and millions more are underinsured and cannot get needed care. A new system does not need to be perfect, it only needs to be vastly superior to the current systems—which is not that difficult.

The American people—consumers, providers and employers—have reason to be motivated for change. If there is a good proposal like Balanced Choice, there is no reason that the change cannot come about. It is just common sense.

Appendices

Appendix A—Essential Balanced Choice Concepts

Essential Balanced Choice Features

Standard Plan
- Small copay or gap payment
- First two visits/year free
- Financial assistance
- Emergency care

Independent Plan
- Greater choice of providers
- Provider able to set fees
- Gap and base payment

Balanced By
- Affordable prices
- Price comparison
- Unbundled choice
- Mandatory Funding Split
- Choice of Plan for both patients and providers
- Independent Plan is reimbursed at less than 100% of the Standard Plan

Quality Maintained By
- Consumer Health Advocacy Organization
- Education is preferred method of regulation
- Medical advisors help patients make choices
- Balanced Choice is a financing system, not a regulatory system

Additional Benefits
- Universal coverage
- Reduced costs for employers
- Eliminates employer responsibility for health care
- Protects employers from future tax increases
- Rapid reimbursement

Balanced Choice is a set of interconnected features that, as a whole, creates an efficient and effective system for financing health care for the entire country. The features are synergistic in that together they are more effective than the sum of the benefits of each feature. While additional features may enhance Balanced Choice, the following Balanced Choice features are considered essential to the Balanced Choice proposal.

Two Plans—Standard Plan and the Independent Plan

Standard Plan	Independent Plan

Standard Plan

This Plan guarantees affordable quality health care.

Small copay or gap payment
On the Standard Plan, copayments are small and gap payments are required for medications, lab tests, and imaging tests.

First two visits/year free
To assure that copays are not an insurmountable barrier to low-income patients, the first two visits per year are free. All providers are able to give low-income patients information about how to obtain financial assistance for additional visits and treatment.

Financial assistance
Low-income patients and patients with catastrophic illnesses are assured financial assistance so that no person needs to forego necessary medical care due to financial hardship.

Emergency care
Because consumers cannot take time to choose between Standard and Independent Plans in emergency situations, all emergency room care is under the Standard Plan.

Independent Plan

This plan allows market forces, not government controls, to contain health care costs.

Greater choice of provider
Patients typically have greater choice of provider under the Independent Plan than the Standard Plan.

Provider able to set fees
Providers have the freedom to set their own fees, and their fees are not controlled by the government

Gap and base payments
Balanced Choice pays a fixed base amount for each category of medication, medical supplies, or some tests. Patients pay the gap between the base amount and the price. Independent Plan patients pay a gap payment for provider visits and procedures. Gap payments maintain consumer cost consciousness

Gap + base = price

The Two Plans Are Balanced By

Affordable prices

Balanced Choice requires that gap payments are affordable, and provides assistance for patients with either low income or catastrophic medical expenses so that no one forgoes necessary medical care due to an inability to pay.

Price comparison

In order for market forces to contain costs, Balanced Choice provides consumers with the information necessary for price comparisons.

Unbundled choice

To the greatest extent practical, choices in Balanced Choice are unbundled and patients are allowed to make one choice at a time.

Mandatory Funding Split

The Balanced Choice Governing Board is required to set Standard Plan reimbursements and Independent Plan reimbursement percentages so that patients and providers voluntarily choose the Standard Plan for 60% of expenditures and voluntarily choose the Independent Plan for 40% of the expenditures.

Choice of Plan for both patients and providers

Balanced Choice allows consumers to change to a provider on a different Plan at any time, and allows providers to change their patients to the Standard Plan at any time or to the Independent Plan with a one-year notice.

Independent Plan is reimbursed at less than 100% of the Standard Plan reimbursement

In order to maintain a clear division between the Standard Plan and the Independent Plan, Balanced Choice reimburses the Independent Plan at less than 100% of the Standard Plan reimbursement.

Quality Is Maintained By

Consumer Health Advocacy Organization

Balanced Choice establishes an independent consumer advocacy organization, the Consumer Health Advocacy Organization. This organization provides consumer education through the *Consumer Health Advocacy Reports*, acts as a watchdog on Balanced Choice, and conducts health care research from the consumer perspective.

Education is the preferred method of regulation

Balanced Choice prefers to solve health care problems through the education of consumers and providers rather than regulation or managed care. Other methods to manage treatment are used only when there is a broad consensus about the need for management, and if there is transparency about the decision making and policies.

Medical advisors help patients make choices

In Balanced Choice, cost information is available when patients meet with their providers so that patients have expert medical advisors to help them make cost decisions based on medical recommendations.

Balanced Choice is a financing system, not a regulatory system

Balanced Choice is a system for financing health care, not regulating health care. The regulation of health care would be conducted independently of Balanced Choice.

Additional Benefits

Universal coverage

Balanced Choice provides universal, birth-to-death, health care coverage regardless of the cause of illness or health care needs.

Reduced costs for employers

A substantial amount of the savings resulting from Balanced Choice is used to reduce employers' costs for health care insurance and the medical portion of workers compensation and automobile insurance.

Eliminates employer responsibility for health care

With Balanced Choice, employers would not be responsible for purchasing or administering health care insurance.

Protects employers from future tax increases for health care

Balanced Choice uses contributions from employers because they are currently paying for much of health care. Employers are guaranteed that their contributions will not be increased when more funding is needed for health care.

Rapid reimbursement

Balanced Choice is required to pay providers within 10 working days of receiving health care claims. There is no need for the traditional 30–60 day delay that has been standard practice in the insurance industry.

Appendix B
Balanced Choice Principles

Balanced Choice is founded on the following guiding principles:

- All residents have a right to quality health care.
- Quality health care systems can be funded by the government, in the same manner that national health care systems are funded in every other industrialized country.
- Employers should not be burdened with the increasingly expensive responsibility of financing the nation's health care system.
- A health care system should be as cost-efficient as possible, spending the maximum amount of dollars on direct patient care without avoidable waste in administrative structures.
- A comprehensive health care system provides benefits for all medically necessary treatment including mental health, pharmaceuticals, and long-term care.
- A health care system should be able to promote prevention, offer early intervention, and provide public education about health and health maintenance for both patients and providers.
- The system should ensure that the nation has a sufficient number of providers and facilities, including emergency and trauma centers.
- Information and financial systems should be easy to use and both consumer and provider-friendly, while reducing paperwork and bureaucracy.
- Efforts to control unavoidable fraud and waste should be cost effective (not cost more than is saved), fully justified, as non-intrusive as possible, non-abrasive, and non-burdensome.
- Balanced Choice is intended to use market forces rather than external controls as much as possible to regulate a system that provides quality health care for all.
- Marketplace dynamics work best when choices for both consumers and providers are not bundled and participants can make as many separate marketplace decisions as possible.
- Unless there are powerful reasons to the contrary, patients should have the power to make health care choices regarding selection, quality, and price.
- A health care system should make it financially possible for patients to maximize their ability to make these choices.
- Regulation, control, and coercion should be minimized.

- Education of consumers and/or providers is the method of first choice to correct problems that cannot be corrected by the market adjustments periodically made by the Balanced Choice Governing Board (BCGB).
- As government regulation becomes more complex and focuses on more details, it is likely also to become more rigid and insensitive, and therefore, government regulation, while necessary and desirable to some degree, should be kept to a minimum and carefully evaluated.
- Providers should have freedom to work outside of a government system, and patients should have freedom to receive treatment outside of a government system.
- The only way to assure that the financial risk of treating illnesses is spread among all citizens is for the government to finance the health care system.
- In order to make the necessary resource balancing adjustments in the system, BCGB must have great flexibility in how it structures the finances of both Plans.
- If there is any need to restrict or ration treatment, it should only be done when there is full public debate and not by hidden treatment guidelines or covert barriers to treatment.
- All health care systems ultimately provide some improved care for those able and willing to pay more for their care. In Balanced Choice, this is accepted as part of the system.
- All health care systems end up providing some free services for those who are unable to pay for their care. In Balanced Choice, this is accepted as part of the system.
- Transparency and disclosure are excellent oversight mechanisms, and all aspects of Balanced Choice should be open to public scrutiny.

Appendix C—Glossary of Terms

Administrative costs: All costs for operations exclusive of disbursements for health care services.

Aggressive managed care: Managed care is intended to guide providers to the most appropriate and effective treatment. Aggressive managed care places a heavy emphasis on lowering cost, and as a result, it has a tendency toward the least expensive treatment options. This usually results in both visible and invisible rationing.

Balanced Choice Governing Board: The governing board appointed by the President of the U.S. and the U.S. Congress to administer Balanced Choice.

Base payment: A designated amount of money that Balanced Choice pays for each service. Actual charges would be greater than the base, and patients would pay the gap between the actual cost of service and the base payment.

Base payment + Gap payment = Cost of Service

Balanced Choice Health Care Fund: The fund that pays for Balanced Choice. It comprises all of the monies collected from federal and state governments and employee and employer contributions. This fund does not include patient out-of-pocket expenses for gap payments or copayments.

Copayments (copays): A patient's share of a health care services payment. The payment is a fixed amount.

Consumer-driven health care: This is a term for a health care financing system that was previously called Medical Savings Accounts. It is a type of health care financing that has a high deductible (usually several thousand dollars) insurance policy that is combined with a Medical Savings Account. Contributions to the Medical Savings Account are tax deductible. In consumer driven health care, decisions about health care—payment, accessibility, treatment, and medication—are made by the patient, or consumer, after consultation with a medical provider. Decisions are based, therefore, on the patient's perspectives and needs.

Consumer Health Advocacy Organization: Suggested name of a Balanced Choice proposed independent consumer organization, which would inform consumers about up-to-date information from scientific research and health concerns, act as a watchdog on Balanced Choice, and conduct health care research from a consumer's perspective.

Diagnostic Related Group (DRG) payments: In this type of funding, a hospital receives a set payment for each patient admitted for each diagnostic group. The payment is based on the average length of stay. These arrangements encourage efficient use of resources. The hospital can save money when an early discharge is appropriate, but it also allows for enough funds for patients to have extended stays when necessary.

Disease management: A treatment service that evaluates and coordinates all aspects of the treatment of a major disease such as diabetes or coronary artery disease. Patients with major illnesses are frequently treated by numerous independent specialists without any single provider coordinating treatment or assuring that the treatment is comprehensive. A disease manager makes sure that treatment is coordinated, that patients are well educated, that duplication is eliminated, and treatment is comprehensive and up-to-date.

Drug formularies: A health care organization's set of internal pharmaceutical regulations regarding which medications are available within the organization, which medications are preferred, how the medications can be obtained, and financial guidelines with limited information about the costs of medications.

Evidence-based medicine: A label that is intended to convey that a medical treatment is based on scientific evidence; it is intended to contrast with the "art" of medicine, which relies heavily on a provider's personal experience and knowledge. There is controversy over how the label is used.

First dollars: When two parties split the payment for services and one party pays a set amount, the party paying the set amount pays the first dollars, and the party paying the remainder pays the last dollars. In insurance, the first dollars are the copayment and in Balanced Choice the first dollars are the base payment. The party who pays last is responsible for price increases and benefits from price decreases. Copayments and base payments are called "first" dollars because as a predetermined amount it can be entered into bookkeeping first before the final price—which may vary—is agreed upon and the "last" dollars are entered.

$$\text{First dollars (a set amount)} + \text{Last dollars} = \text{Price}$$

Functional market: A functional market has dynamics that press for higher quality, greater accessibility, and lower prices. Functional market is intended to contrast with using the term "market" to describe any situation in which money is transferred, regardless of its effects on quality, accessibility, or prices. In order to create a functional health care market, Balanced Choice requires the following market principles:

1. Consumers have unbundled choices of goods and services.
2. Consumers have easy access to the information they need to make informed choices.
3. Choices are affordable for a large portion of the market.
4. Price comparison is easy.
5. Providers are free to set fees that the market will support.
6. Consumers and providers are free to change choices.
7. Consumers, not employers or insurance companies, make purchasing choices.
8. Cost is contained by the cost consciousness of consumers.

Gap payments: Payments a patient makes to cover the difference (or gap) between a set base payment made by Balanced Choice funds and the actual cost of a service. Economically, the gap payment is the last dollars, which means the patient is responsible for cost increases and benefits from cost reductions.

$$\text{Base payment} + \text{Gap payment} = \text{Cost of service}$$

Gross Domestic Product (GDP): The total value of all goods and services produced annually by everyone in the United States. The figure amounts do not include losses or expenditures.

Independent Plan: One of two options of payment Plans in Balanced Choice. In this Plan, providers set any fee they choose. Balanced Choice funds pay an established base payment (less than with the Standard Plan) and patients pay the gap. Medications, imaging tests, and lab tests also require a gap payment.

Independent Plan reimbursement percentage: The percentage of the Standard Plan Reimbursement schedule that Independent Plan providers receive from Balanced Choice. This amount is always less than 100%, and it may be adjusted by the Balanced Choice Governing Board in order to maintain the Mandatory Funding Split.

Insurance-driven health care: Describes health care when insurance companies and entities that act like traditional insurance pay the majority of the cost of health care. Characteristics of insurance-driven systems are that the insurance company pays the last dollar, consumers are shielded from full cost consciousness, and consumers are divided into different risk pools.

Invisible rationing: A process in which consumers are denied health care options without being informed about the potential benefits of more extensive treatment or alternative treatments.

Last dollars: When two parties split the payment for services and one party pays a set amount, the party paying the set amount pays the first dollars, and the party paying the remainder pays the last dollars. In insurance, the first dollars are the copayment and in Balanced Choice the first dollars are the base payment. The party who pays last is responsible for price increases and benefits from price decreases. Copayments and base payments are called "first" dollars because as a predetermined amount it can be entered into bookkeeping first before the final price—which may vary—is agreed upon and the "last" dollars are entered.

First Dollars (a set amount) + Last dollars = Price

Managed care: A system in which a third party intervenes in the physician-patient (first and second parties) relationship with policies and procedures that are intended to lower the cost of treatment. The third party benefits from a reduction in the cost of treatment.

Mandatory Funding Split: The Balanced Choice Governing Board is required to set Standard Plan reimbursements and Independent Plan reimbursement percentages so that patients and providers voluntarily choose the Standard Plan for 60% of expenditures and voluntarily choose the Independent Plan for 40% of the expenditures.

Market-based system: Economic term referring to an American-style system that has competition, allows consumers choice of goods and services, allows providers to set fees, and responds to supply and demand factors.

Medical cost offset: Refers to the amount that the cost of future medical services is reduced as a result of providing mental health services.

Medical Savings Account (MSA): A tax-exempt personal savings account designated to pay for medical expenses. The savings account is combined with a high deductible (several thousand dollars) catastrophic insurance policy. A consumer contributes money and spends it on medical bills up to the limit of the deductible. Because consumers spend their own money, they are inclined to make treatment decisions that consider financial ramifications.

Monopoly: An economic term denoting a system in which one entity can control the available production of goods or services. This eliminates competition because the entity has the power to control availability, quality, and price. As a result, availability and quality decline, and prices rise.

Monopsony: An economic term denoting a system in which one entity controls all of the consumers. While this system can demand lower prices, it also eliminates competitive forces because producers of services cannot offer different services at different rates to different customers. As a result, prices decline, but quality and accessibility also decline.

National Health Expenditures (NHE): An estimate by the Centers for Medicaid and Medicare Studies of the amount that is spent on health care in the United States annually.

Pharmacy tiers: A common arrangement for pricing of medications in which generics are on the first tier, brands preferred because of preferential pricing arrangements with the managed care company are on a second tier, and the non-preferred brand names are on the third tier. The first tier has the lowest copayment, the second tier has a higher copayment, and the third tier has the highest copayment.

Proprietary guidelines/rules/information: Indicates that the information, guidelines, or rules are owned by a person, group, or company and, as such, are confidential and are usually withheld or hidden from the public.

Reference pricing: A method of pricing medications that is used in Europe, and which is similar to Balanced Choice. Categories of medication are reimbursed with a base payment (reference price) for each category and patients pay the gap.

Reimbursement schedule adjustment: Changes in the Standard Plan reimbursement schedule and the Independent Plan reimbursement percentage made by the Balanced Choice Governing Board in order to entice consumers and providers to choose health care plans in a manner that results in the 60/40 Mandatory Funding Split.

Single payer system: Plan that would provide health care coverage to everyone, funded by taxes and managed by a government agency that would set provider fees. A single payer (the government) would replace health insurance and multiple other health care entities that currently pay providers' fees.

Standard Plan: One of two options of payment plans in Balanced Choice. In this Plan, fees are set by the Balanced Choice Governing Board in much the same way as Medicare. Patients usually have a small copayment and providers receive the remainder of the reimbursement from the Balanced Choice. The Standard Plan covers all emergencies. Medications, imaging tests, and lab tests usually require a gap payment. Balanced Choice assists low-income consumers and patients with catastrophic medical expenses with their copayments and gap payments.

Standard Plan reimbursement schedule: A list of the amount that Balanced Choice will reimburse providers for each treatment code.

Stakeholders: Entities (people or groups) whose interests are influenced—at stake—by policies and decisions being addressed.

Third-party payer: Bills are paid by an entity or "party" not involved in either providing or receiving services (the patient is the first party and the provider is the second party). For example, when an insurance company rather than the patient pays a doctor's fee, the insurance company is the third party.

Unbundled choices: Individual choices in contrast to combining many choices in packaged plans.

Underinsured: Refers to health insurance that either does not cover all necessary health care or does not provide sufficient reimbursement to make health care affordable.

Uninsurable: Refers to a situation in which insurance companies refuse to provide health care coverage, typically because a patient has an illness that presents a risk to the insurance company that medical bills will be costly.

Universal coverage: In a given population, such as the United States, everyone has the financial assistance needed for necessary health care services.

Universal health care vouchers: A proposal for a federally funded voucher system that could be used by consumers toward the purchase of health insurance. In this system, those who could afford and who wanted better coverage would upgrade with personal money.

Utilization review: A process in which a managed care company reviews treatment decisions and treatment plans in order to make decisions about which treatments and how much treatment is worth the cost.

Endnotes

Preface

1. Miller, I. J. (1996). Time-limited brief therapy has gone too far: The result is invisible rationing. *Professional Psychology: Research and Practice, 27(6),* 567–576; Miller, I. J. (1996). Some "short-term therapy values" are a formula for invisible rationing. *Professional Psychology: Research and Practice, 27(6),* 577–582; and Miller, I. J. (1996). Ethical and liability issues concerning invisible rationing. *Professional Psychology: Research and Practice, 27(6),* 583–587.

2. 1997 American Psychiatric Association Convention, San Diego, CA. Presidential Issues Media Briefing, "Managed care methods based on fictional research," Ivan J. Miller, Ph.D., and Harold Eist, M.D. President of the American Psychiatric Association with commentary by Karen Shore, Ph.D., President, National Coalition of Mental Health Professionals and Consumers, Inc.; Dorothy Cantor, Ph.D., Past President, American Psychological Association; Betty Phillips, Ph.D., President, Clinical Social Work Federation; and Stanley Moldawsky, Ph.D., American Psychological Association, President of the Division of Independent Practice.

3. Miller, I. J. (1996). Managed care is harmful to outpatient mental health services: A call for accountability. *Professional Psychology: Research and Practice, 27(4),* 349–363.

4. Anderson, K. (1997). "Collusive behavior in the managed care industry." This "white paper" and a supplement prepared by I. J. Miller were submitted to Department of Justice with a follow-up meeting with the Antitrust Division of the DOJ. This report described anti-competitive behavior in the managed mental health care industry including discussions of monopsony and managed care as an economic system.

Chapter 1. Balanced Choice: A Health Care Security System

5. Families USA. (2004). One in three: Non-elderly Americans without health insurance, 2002–2003. Publication Number 04–104. Washington, DC: Author.

6. Reinhardt, U. E., Hussey, P. S., & Anderson, G. F. (2003). U.S. health care spending in an international context. *Health Affairs, 23(3),* 10–25. Cites that U.S. spends $4,887 per person annually and the next greatest expenditure is Switzerland spending $3,332 based on Organization for Economic Cooperation and Development (OECD) 2002 data and reported in U.S. dollar purchasing-power parities.

7. Hussey, P. S., Anderson, G. F., Osborn, R., Feek, C., McLaughlin, V., Millar, J., & Epstein, A. (2004). How does the quality of care compare in five countries? *Health Affairs, 23(3),* 89–99. This article, combined with data from Reinhardt, Hussey, & Anderson (2003), op. cit., regarding the comparative expenses of Australia, United Kingdom, New Zealand, and Canada, shows that the U.S. health care systems have quality problems.

Chapter 2. Making Sense of Health Care Economics
8. Richmond, J. B. & Fein, R. (2005). *The health care mess: How we got into it and what it will take to get out.* Cambridge: Harvard University Press.
9. Ibid.
10. Blair, R. D. & Harrison, J. L. (1950). Antitrust policy and monopsony. *Cornell Law Review, 76*:297–340.
11. Gilmer, T. & Kronick, R. (2005). It's the premiums, stupid: projections of the uninsured through 2013. Health Affairs, *W5,* 143–151.
12. Families USA. (2004). One in Three: Non-Elderly Americans Without Health Insurance, 2002–2003. Publication Number 04–104. Washington, DC: Author. For all or part of 2002 and 2003, 81.8 million people were without health insurance, and the U.S. population was estimated at 290 million according to the *New York Times Almanac* (Wright, 2004).
13. Kleinke, J. D. (2001). *Oxymorons: The myth of a U.S. health care system.* San Francisco: Josey-Bass.
14. Reinhardt, U. E., Hussey, P. S., & Anderson, G. F. (2004). U.S. health care spending in an international context. *Health Affairs, 23(3),* 10–25.
15. Hussey, P. S., Anderson, G. F., Osborn, R., Feek, C., McLaughlin, V., Millar, J., & Epstein, A. (2004). How does the quality of care compare in five countries? *Health Affairs, 23(3)*, 89–99.
16. Ibid.

Chapter 4. An Outline for Financing Balanced Choice
17. Reinhardt, U. E., Hussey, P. S. & Anderson, G. F. (2004). U.S. health care spending in an international context, *Health Affairs, 23(3)*, 10–25.
18. Woolhandler, S., Campbell, T., & Himmelstein, D. U. (2003). Costs of health care administration in the United States and Canada. *New England Journal of Medicine, 349,* 768–775. U.S. administrative costs accounted for 31% of health care spending and Canadian administrative costs accounted for 16.7% of health care spending in 1987. This is a 14.3% difference. According to National Health Care Expenditures Projected Aggregate by Source of Funds compiled by the Centers for Medicare and Medicaid

Services (2005) health care spending for 2004 was $1,805 billion, which was multiplied by 14.3% to obtain a difference of $258 billion.

19. Hadley, J. & Holahan, J. (2003). How much medical care do the uninsured use, and who pays for it? *Health Affairs, W3,* 66–81.

20. Hadley, J. & Holahan, J. (2003). Covering the uninsured: How much would it cost? *Health Affairs, W3,* 250–265.

21. Hadley and Holahan, op.cit., reported that in 2001 there were 41 million uninsured and in 2004 there were 44 million uninsured. The 6% figure was raised to 6.4% to adjust for the increase in the number of uninsured, and this was multiplied by the NHE for 2004 of $1.805 billion.

22. National Health Care Expenditures Projected Aggregate by Source of Funds compiled by the Centers for Medicare and Medicaid Services. (2005).

23. Himmelstein, D. U., Warren, E., Thorne, D., & Woolhandler, S. (2005). Illness and injury as contributors to bankruptcy. *Health Affairs, W5,* 63–73.

Chapter 6. The Provider-Friendly Experience in Balanced Choice

24. I have some personal experience to bring to the provider's perspective. I have been operating a clinical psychology practice that has no contracts with insurance or managed care for 11 years. In addition, for 11 years I have been the founder and president of the Boulder Psychotherapists' Guild, a group that now has 78 independent psychotherapists who are interested in increasing the number of self-pay clients. We are contracting directly with patients, not insurance companies. Many of our patients have an insurance plan that would pay for much of their treatment if they stayed in network, but they think it is worth paying a higher amount or the whole amount to see an independent, out-of-network psychotherapist. We have found that many patients are willing to pay a higher amount if they think they are getting more benefits.

25. Waters, W. C. III. (1999) *The grand disguise: A practicing doctor's analysis of healthcare.* Atlanta: Eklektik Press.

Chapter 7. A Balanced Choice Pharmacy Plan

26. Families USA. (2004). Sticker shock: rising prescription drug prices for seniors. Washington DC: Author. Of 30 brand-name drugs most frequently used by the elderly, the cost of the 26 that have been on the market for over three years rose at 3.6 times the rate of inflation from 1/01–1/04. A review of these 26 in the *Physician's Desk Reference,* 2004, reveals that at least 22 have competitors.

27. Families USA. (2003). Out of bounds. Washington DC: Author.

28. Families USA. (2005). The choice: Health care for people or drug industry profits. Publication No. 05–104, Washington DC: Families USA.
29. Kanavos, P. and U. E. Reinhardt. (2003). Reference pricing for drugs: Is it compatible with U.S. health care? *Health Affairs, 22(3)*, 16–30.
30. Ibid.
31. McCloskey, A. (2000). Cost overdose: Growth in drug spending for the elderly, *1992–2010*. Washington DC: Families USA.
32. Baker, D. (2006). The excess cost of the Medicare drug benefit, Washington, DC: Institute for America's Future Center for Economic and Policy Research.
33. Kravitz, R. L. & Change, S. (2005). Promise and perils for patients and physicians, *New England Journal of Medicine, 353*, 2735–2739.
34. Families USA. (2005). Pick a plan: The new CMS drug benefit game for seniors, Washington DC: Author.
35. Families USA. (2005). Gearing up: States face the new Medicare law. The holes in Part D: Gaps in the new Medicare drug benefit (Part 1 of 2), Washington DC: Author.
36. Families USA. (2004). The Medicare road show. Washington DC: Author. Families USA explains that in the model program there is a $35/mo. premium, $250 deductible, insurance coverage of 75% for expenses between $250 and $2,250, and a $2,850 gap in coverage for expenses between $2,250 and $5,100.
37. Kaiser Family Foundation. (2006). Selected findings on seniors' views of the Medicare prescription drug benefit. Publication #7463. Washington, DC: Author.

Chapter 8. Science, Education, and Consumer Advocacy

38. Millenson, M. L. (1997). *Demanding medical excellence: Doctors and accountability in the information age.* Chicago: University of Chicago Press.
39. In my practice as a psychologist, I frequently hear stories demonstrating the power of the Internet. Illness and interactions with the medical community are emotional issues that patients discuss in therapy. It is common for my patients to tell me that they have researched either their illness or the illness of a family member on the Internet. Often they report discussing this research with their provider. At times it affects their choice of treatment. Other times, they report that the provider was interested in personally learning more about something that came from the Internet. Without any regulatory intervention, this avenue holds promise for increasing the adoption of evidence-based medicine.

40. The proposed publication, *Consumer Health Care Reports*, is not endorsed by or associated with Consumers Union or its publication *Consumer Reports.*

Chapter 9. More Features and Innovation

41. McGinnis, J. M. & Foege, W. H. (1993). Actual causes of death in the United States. *Journal of the American Medical Association 270*, 2207–12. The ten major causes of death were identified as tobacco, diet, activity patterns, alcohol, microbial agents, toxic agents, firearms, sexual behavior, motor vehicles, and illicit drugs. All but microbial agents, toxic agents, and arguably firearms are modifiable by behavior changes.
42. American Psychological Association. (2006). Medical Cost Offset. http://www.apa.org/practice/offset3.html Washington, DC: Author.
43. Schlesinger, H. J., Mumford, E., Glass, G. V., Patrick, C., & Sharfstein, S. (1983). Mental health treatment and medical care utilization in a fee-for-service system: Outpatient mental health treatment following the onset of a chronic illness. *American Journal of Public Health, 73*, 422–429.
44. Hay Group, Washington DC survey, funded by the National Alliance for the Mentally Ill, the National Association of Psychiatric Health Systems, and the Association of Behavioral Group Practices 5/7/98. It found funding for mental health services was decreased 54% from 1988 to 1997 (www.nami.org). Psychotherapy Finances. (1996). Practice Issues: Employers are slashing behavioral health expenses. *Psychotherapy Finances 22 (10)*, p. 1. This article reported that in a Foster Higgins employer survey, the percent of employers' insurance costs that funded mental health services declined from 9% in 1989 to 4% in 1996.
45. Sharkey, Joe. (1994). *Bedlam: Greed, profiteering, and fraud in a mental health system gone crazy.* New York: St. Martin's Press,.

Chapter 10. Health Care Insurance is Obsolete

46. Top Industries Giving to Members of Congress 2004 and 2006 The Center for Responsive Politics, www.opensecrets.org. Washington, DC: Author.
47. American Psychological Association. (2006). Medical Cost Offset. http://www.apa.org/practice/offset3.html. Washington, DC: Author
48. Holstein, Russell M. (2004). Triage as treatment: Phantom mental health services at Kaiser-Permanente. *Independent Practitioner, 24(2)*. http://www.division42.org/MembersArea/IPfiles/IPSpring04/TOC.html. Washington, DC: American Psychological Association.

Chapter 11. Patching-Up Insurance-Driven Health Care

49. Miller, I. J. (1996). Time-limited brief therapy has gone too far: The result is invisible rationing. *Professional Psychology: Research and Practice, 27(6)*, 567–576; Miller, I. J. (1996). Some "short-term therapy values" are a formula for invisible rationing. *Professional Psychology: Research and Practice, 27(6)*, 577–582; Miller, I. J. (1996). Ethical and liability issues concerning invisible rationing. *Professional Psychology: Research and Practice, 27(6)*, 583–587; Miller, I. J. (1996). Managed care is harmful to outpatient mental health services: A call for accountability. *Professional Psychology: Research and Practice, 27(4)*, 349–363.

50. Negotiated discounts are generally closely guarded proprietary information. To obtain this estimate I examined my family's 28 insurance claims for 2004. Each insurance claim was processed through Sloan's Lake Insurance, which has Colorado's largest PPO network (www. SloansLake.com). The claims listed the amount charged to individuals who are not affiliated with an insurance company and the amount that this charge was reduced because the provider had contracted with Sloans Lake. The adjusted discounts on the claims ranged from 0% to 100%, and most discounts were near the mean, 39%. A cash-paying patient or uninsured patient would have been charged 64% more than my family paid due to the negotiated discounts that came from the affiliation with Sloans Lake. Because Sloans Lake is the largest PPO in Colorado, the adjusted discounts can be considered common.

Chapter 12. Balanced Choice Compared to Single Payer

51. Hussey, P. S., Anderson, G. F., Osborn, R., Feek, C., McLaughlin, V., Millar, J., & Epstein, A. (2004). How does the quality of care compare in five countries? *Health Affairs, 23(3)*, 89–99.

52. Woolhandler, S. & Himmelstein, D. U. (2002). Paying for national health insurance—and not getting it. *Health Affairs, 21(4)*, 88–98.

Chapter 13. Balanced Choice has Solid Advantages: A Reply to Skepticism

53. Kamal-Bahl, S. & Briesacher, B. (2004). How do incentive-based formularies influence drug selection and spending for hypertension? *Health Affairs, 23(1)*, 227–236.

54. Robinson, J. C. (2003). Hospital tiers in health insurance: Balancing consumer choice with financial incentives. *Health Affairs, W3*, 135–146.

Index

Printed in the United States
58243LVS00004B/157-168

9 781425 956707